Introducing Palliative Care

Second edition

Robert Twycross DM, FRCP, FRCR

Macmillan Clinical Reader in Palliative Medicine,
Oxford University
Consultant Physician, Sir Michael Sobell House,
Churchill Hospital, Oxford
Senior Research Fellow, St Peter's College, Oxford
Director, WHO Collaborating Centre for Palliative
Cancer Care, Oxford
Chairman, International School for Cancer Care

RADCLIFFE MEDICAL PRESS
OXFORD AND NEW YORK

©1997 Robert Twycross

Radcliffe Medical Press Ltd
18 Marcham Road, Abingdon, Oxon, OX14 1AA, UK

Radcliffe Medical Press, Inc.
141 Fifth Avenue, New York, NY 10010, USA

First edition 1995
Reprinted 1996

British Library Cataloguing in Publication Data
A catalogue record for this book is available from the British Library.

ISBN 1 85775 260 0

Library of Congress Cataloging-in-Publication Data is available.

CJ

Typeset by AMA Graphics Limited, Preston
Printed and bound in Great Britain by Biddles Ltd, Guildford and King's Lynn

Contents

Preface

This book represents a further stage in the evolution of a set of lecture notes originally prepared over a decade ago for clinical students of the Oxford University Medical School attending a five day course at Sir Michael Sobell House on 'Care of the Patient with Advanced Cancer'. Several other centres both in the UK and in other countries have also made use of them, in some cases translating them into the local language. Because of the continued interest in the lecture notes, they have been revised and are being published professionally in a format which is easier to handle and which will facilitate their use as a course manual.

Specialist palliative care services are often focused on the care of patients with endstage cancer. The same is true of this book. The general principles and most of the details, however, are applicable to patients dying from other progressive incurable disorders. The content is inevitably selective, notably in relation to symptom management. The book also reflects an emphasis on 'whole person' care, ethics, communication skills, coping with loss, as well as providing an introduction to pain and symptom management.

When compiling a book of this nature, it is necessary to acknowledge many people and sources, some long forgotten. One is reminded of the old saying that, 'There is nothing new under the sun'. To the anonymous teachers from the past, I express my gratitude. In the pages devoted to communication and breaking bad news, the perceptive reader may well see the more obvious shadows of Ivan Lichter, Susan Le Poidevin, Robert Buckman and Peter Maguire. David Frampton made many useful suggestions, as did Gilly Burn, Karen Jenns, Andrew Wilcock and Angela Williams.

The help of course tutors, past and present, is also acknowledged. These include Jennifer Barraclough, John Barton, Ruben Bild, David Cook, Ann Couldrick, Ginny Dunn, Michael Minton, Sue Palmer, Marilyn Relf, Victoria Slater, Rosalyn Staveley, and Averil Stedeford. Where a sole or prime author is still clearly identifiable, this is acknowledged in the text.

Robert Twycross
January 1997

Drug names

For some drugs marketed in the UK, the International Nonproprietary Name (INN) differs from the British Approved Name (BAN). From January 1998, the use of BANs will be discontinued and all drugs marketed in the UK will be known by their INN.

More than 40 drugs have a BAN which is different from their corresponding INN; those relevant to palliative care are listed below.

BAN	INN
Adrenaline	Epinephrine
Amylobarbitone	Amobarbital
Bendrofluazide	Bendroflumethiazide
Benzhexol	Trihexyphenidyl
Benztropine	Benzatropine
Chlorpheniramine	Chlorphenamine
Dicyclomine	Dicycloverine
Dimethicone	Dimeticone
Frusemide	Furosemide
Hexamine hippurate	Methenamine hippurate
Indomethacin	Indometacin
Lignocaine	Lidocaine
Methotrimeprazine	Levomepromazine
Noradrenaline	Norepinephrine
Oestradiol	Estradiol
Oxethazaine	Oxetacaine
Phenobarbitone	Phenobarbital
Stilboestrol	Diethylstilbestrol
Trimeprazine	Alimemazine

Differences also exist between INNs and adopted names in the USA (USANs).

INN	USAN
Dimeticone	Simethicone
Dextropropoxyphene	Propoxyphene
Glycopyrronium	Glycopyrrolate
Paracetamol	Acetaminophen
Pethidine	Meperidine

Note also that

● diamorphine (available only in the UK and Canada) = di-acetylmorphine = heroin

● hyoscine = scopolamine

● liquid paraffin = mineral oil.

All the drugs referred to in *Introducing Palliative Care* are not universally available. Please check with your own National Formulary or drug compendium if in doubt.

List of abbreviations

General

BNF	British National Formulary
BP	British Pharmacopoeia
IASP	International Association for the Study of Pain
UK	United Kingdom
USA	United States of America
USP	United States Pharmacopoeia
WHO	World Health Organization

Medical

CNS	central nervous system
COPD	chronic obstructive pulmonary disease
COX	cyclo-oxygenase
CSF	cerebrospinal fluid
CT	computed tomography
5HT	5-hydroxytryptamine (serotonin)
H_1, H_2	histamine type 1, type 2 receptors
MAOI(s)	mono-amine oxidase inhibitor(s)
MRI	magnetic resonance imaging
NMDA	N-methyl D-aspartate
NSAID(s)	nonsteroidal anti-inflammatory drug(s)
PCA	patient controlled analgesia
PG(s)	prostaglandin(s)
SSRI(s)	selective serotonin re-uptake inhibitor(s)

Drug administration

b.d.	twice daily; alternative, b.i.d.
ED	epidural

IM	intramuscular
IT	intrathecal
IV	intravenous
m/r	modified release; alternative, slow release
nocte	at bedtime
o.d.	daily, once a day
p.c.	post cebus, after meals
PO	per os, by mouth
PR	per rectum, by rectum
q.d.s.	four times a day (per 24 h); alternative, q.i.d.
q4h, q6h	every 4 hours, every 6 hours etc.
SC	subcutaneous
SL	sublingual
stat	immediately
t.d.s.	three times a day (per 24 h); alternative, t.i.d.

Units

cm	centimetre(s)
Gy	Gray(s), a measure of radiation
g	gram(s)
h	hour(s)
Hg	mercury
IU	international unit(s)
kg	kilogram(s)
l	litre(s)
mcg	microgram(s)
mEq	milli-equivalent(s)
mg	milligram(s)
ml	millilitre(s)
mm	millimetre(s)
mmol	millimole(s)
min	minute(s)

PART ONE

General Topics

Fatal statistics · Palliative care
A typical palliative care service
Dying at home
Ethical considerations · Hope

Fatal statistics

Cancer is common.

One third of the population in the UK develops cancer.

One quarter of the population in the UK dies of cancer.

These figures are true for all developed countries. The incidence has increased considerably over the last 30 years. It is still increasing because of

- tobacco smoking
- an ageing population.

Despite these gloomy figures, it is important to have a balanced view of cancer because

- some cancers can be cured, possibly as many as one third
- even if incurable, people may survive for many years.

For example, 16% of a group of patients with colorectal cancer noted to have a solitary hepatic metastasis at the time of the initial laparotomy survived 5 years.[1]

Further, it has been shown in breast cancer patients that[2]

- a fighting spirit or denial results in a better prognosis
- fatalism or helplessness/hopelessness results in a worse prognosis.

Palliative care

Palliative is derived from a Latin word 'pallium', meaning a cloak or cover. Thus, in palliative care, symptoms are 'cloaked' with treatments whose primary or sole aim is to promote patient comfort.

Definition and scope

Palliative care is the active total care of patients and their families by a multiprofessional team at a time when the patient's disease is no longer responsive to curative treatment and life expectancy is relatively short (Figure 1.1). It responds to physical, psychological, social and spiritual needs, and extends if necessary to support in bereavement (Figure 1.2). The goal of palliative care is to provide support and care for patients in the last phases of the disease so that they can live as fully and comfortably as possible.

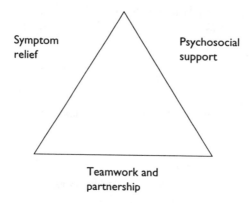

Figure 1.1 Three essential components of palliative care.

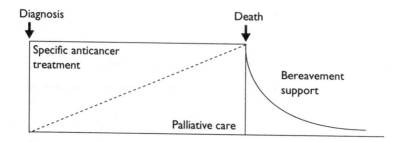

Figure 1.2 Diagram to show the relationship between anticancer treatment and palliative care over time.

Although sometimes described as 'low tech and high touch', palliative care is not intrinsically against medical technology. Rather it seeks to ensure that compassion and not science is the controlling force in patient care. High tech investigations and treatments are used only when their benefits clearly outweigh any potential burdens.

Palliative care includes rehabilitation. It seeks to help patients achieve and maintain their maximum potential physically, psychologically, socially and spiritually, however limited these have become as a result of disease progression. Palliative care

- affirms life and regards dying as a normal process
- neither hastens nor postpones death
- provides relief for patients from pain and other distressing symptoms
- integrates psychological, social and spiritual aspects of care so that patients may come to terms with their own death as fully and constructively as they can
- offers a support system to help patients live as actively and creatively as possible until death
- offers a support system to help families cope during the patient's illness and in bereavement
- is often called 'hospice care', particularly in the UK.

Teamwork

Palliative care is best administered by a group of people working as a team. The team is collectively concerned with the total wellbeing of the patient and family. In practice, some or all of the following will be involved

- doctor(s) and nurses (essential core clinical team)
- physiotherapist, occupational therapist, and other specific therapists
- social worker, chaplain/priest/rabbi and/or other advisers
- volunteers.

Because there is an overlap of roles, co-ordination is an important part of teamwork. Conflict inevitably erupts from time to time in a team of highly motivated, skilled professionals. One of the challenges of teamwork is how to handle conflict constructively and creatively.

Partnership

The essence of palliative care is *partnership* between the caring team and the patient and family. Partnership requires mutual respect. Partnership and respect are manifested by

- courtesy in behaviour
- politeness in speech
- not patronizing
- being honest
- listening
- explaining
- agreeing priorities and goals
- discussing treatment options
- accepting treatment refusal.

Taken collectively, the above list provides the basis for an individual approach to care.

'Care begins when difference is recognized. I reserve the name "caregivers" for the people who are willing to listen to ill persons and to respond to their individual experiences. Caring has nothing to do with categories. When the caregiver communicates to the ill person that she cares about the patient's uniqueness, she makes the person's life meaningful.'[3]

Quality of life

'Quality of life is what a person says it is.'

It is often said that the goal of palliative care is the highest possible quality of life for both patient and family. Quality of life refers to subjective satisfaction experienced and/or expressed by an individual; it relates to and is influenced by all the dimensions of personhood – physical, psychological, social and spiritual.

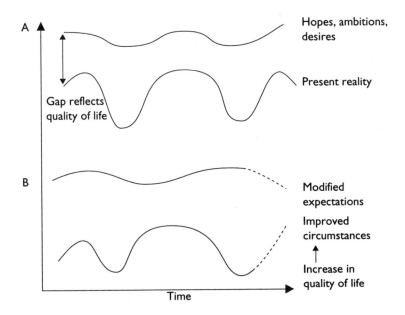

Figure 1.3 A: a representation of the gap between reality and hopes. B: improvement in quality of life represents either a reduction in expectations or a change in present reality.[4]

There is good quality of life when the aspirations of an individual are matched and fulfilled by present experience. There is poor quality of life when there is a wide divergence between aspirations and present experience.[4] To improve quality of life, it is necessary to narrow the gap between aspirations and what is possible (Figure 1.3).

Thus, a tetraplegic ex-gymnastics instructor is able to say, 'The quality of my life is excellent, though to see me you wouldn't believe it. I've come to terms with my loss and discovered the powers of my mind.' And a 30 year-old man dying of disseminated osteosarcoma complicated by paraplegia comments, 'The last year of my life has been the best.'

Quality of life scores tend to be flawed because they measure only selected aspects and not global subjective satisfaction.[5–7]

A typical palliative care service

Although focusing on home care, most palliative care services in the UK offer a range of services

● specialist home care nurses

- medical consultations:
  at home with the general practitioner
  in other wards and hospitals
- outpatient clinics
- day care
- inpatient care
- bereavement support
- education (generally)
- research (sometimes).

Clinical services are directed by a medical director/consultant physician and a matron/senior nurse. Typically, about 95% of patients have cancer. Although there is a provider contract with one or more health authority, a variable amount of money needs to be raised annually to make ends meet – anything from 30–70% of the total cost of the service.

Home care

Specialist home care nurses (often called Macmillan nurses) liaise with the primary health care team and offer advice on treatment and care. Because they provide support for the whole family, more patients are able to remain at home until death.

Day care

A day centre receives 10–15 patients a day. Patients are driven to and from the centre by volunteers. Patients attend for social support and to give the family a break. Medical and nursing care is also available. Services include bathing, hairdressing, manicure, chiropody and massage. The day centre enables many patients to remain at home for much longer than would otherwise be possible.

Patients attending a day centre often find new meaning and purpose in living as they make new friends, explore opportunities for creative expression, and enjoy cultural activities together.

Inpatient care

Patients are admitted for symptom management, for family relief (respite) or to die. About half of all admissions end with the patient returning home or to relatives. A high nurse–patient ratio is maintained because the physical and psychological needs of the patients are often considerable.

Rehabilitation is facilitated by an occupational therapist and a physiotherapist. Inpatients are encouraged to make use of the facilities of the day centre. The median length of stay is typically 8–10 days.

Bereavement support

This may be provided by trained volunteers under the supervision of a social worker. They offer support to a number of bereaved relatives and other key carers. Support may also be continued after bereavement by the home care nurses.

Voluntary help

The support provided by a specialist palliative care service is enhanced by volunteers who are involved in many aspects of the care. Volunteers receive initial and continuing inservice training.

Education and research

Education is an important aspect of palliative care. Various courses give opportunities for other health care professionals to learn how to care better for dying patients.

Research is important if the care of dying patients is to be improved further. It is time-consuming and costly, and is undertaken by only a small number of units.

Dying at home

Most people, if given the opportunity, would choose to die at home rather than in the alien environment of a hospital. With good support services, high quality care is often possible at home and may well be more appropriate for the patient and family.

Prerequisites for good home care

Any or all of the following may be required

- primary health care team:
    general practitioner
    community nurse
- community care services
- specialist support team:
    home care nurse
    palliative care physician
    social worker
    clinical psychologist/psychotherapist
    occupational therapist
- priest/rabbi etc.
- friends or volunteers to sit with the patient while the key carer goes shopping or has time off
- day care
- outpatient evaluation
- night nurses
- short periods of inpatient care:
    for symptom management
    to give the family a rest (respite).

Ethical considerations

The ethics of palliative care are those of medicine in general. Doctors have a dual responsibility, namely to preserve life and to relieve suffering. At the end of life, relief of suffering is of even greater importance as preserving life becomes increasingly impossible.

Four cardinal principles[8]

- patient autonomy (respect for the patient as a person)
- beneficence (do good)
- nonmaleficence (minimize harm)
- justice (fair use of available resources).

The four cardinal principles need to be applied against a background of

- respect for life
- acceptance of the ultimate inevitability of death.

In practice, these comprise three dichotomies which need to be applied in a balanced manner. Thus

- the potential benefits of treatment must be balanced against the potential burdens
- striving to preserve life but, when biologically futile, providing comfort in dying
- individual needs are balanced against those of society.

Appropriate treatment

All patients must die eventually. Part of the art of medicine is to decide when sustaining life is essentially futile and, therefore, when to allow death to occur without further impediment. Thus, in palliative care, the primary aim of treatment is not to prolong life but to make the life which remains as comfortable and as meaningful as possible.

A doctor is not obliged legally or ethically to preserve life 'at all costs'. Rather, life should be sustained when from a biological point of view it is sustainable. Priorities change when a patient is clearly dying. There is no obligation to employ treatments if their use can best be described as prolonging the process of dying. A doctor has neither a duty nor the right to prescribe a lingering death.

It is not a question of to treat or not to treat but what is the most appropriate treatment given the patient's biological prospects and his personal and social circumstances? Appropriate treatment for an acutely ill patient may be inappropriate in the dying (Figures 1.4 and 1.5).

Nasogastric tubes, IV infusions, antibiotics, cardiac resuscitation, and artificial respiration are all primarily support measures for use in acute or acute-on-chronic illnesses to assist a patient through the initial crisis towards recovery of health. To use such measures in patients who are close to death and in whom there is no expectation of a return to health is generally inappropriate (and therefore bad medicine).

Medical care is a continuum, ranging from complete cure at one end to symptom relief at the other. Many types of treatment span the entire spectrum, notably radiotherapy and, to a lesser extent, chemotherapy and surgery. It is

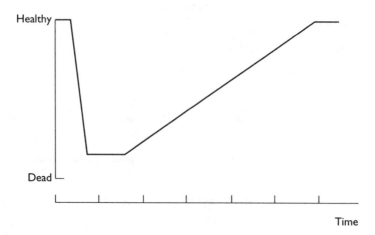

Figure 1.4   A graphical representation of acute illness. Biological prospects are generally good. Acute resuscitative measures are important and enable the patient to survive the initial crisis. Recovery is aided by the natural forces of healing; rehabilitation is completed by the patient on his own, without continued medical support.

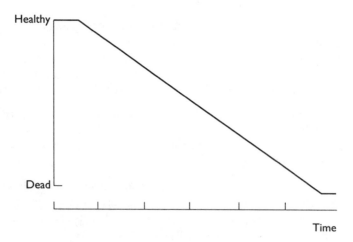

Figure 1.5   A graphical representation of terminal illness. Biological prospects progressively worsen. Acute and terminal illnesses are therefore distinct pathophysiological entities. Therapeutic interventions which can best be described as prolonging the distress of dying are futile and inappropriate.

important to keep the therapeutic aim clearly in mind with any form of treatment. In deciding what is appropriate, the key points are

- the patient's biological prospects
- the therapeutic aim and benefits of each treatment
- the adverse effects of treatment
- the need not to prescribe a lingering death.

Although the possibility of unexpected improvement or recovery should not be ignored, there are many occasions when it is appropriate to 'give death a chance'.

As a person becomes terminally ill, or severely limited physically and mentally as a result of senile decay, his interest in hydration and nutrition often becomes minimal. Because the natural outcome of both incurable progressive disease and advanced senility is death, these are circumstances in which it is wrong to force a patient to accept food and fluid. The patient's disinterest or positive disinclination should be seen as part of the process of letting go.

Hope

'Hope is an expectation greater than zero of achieving a goal.'

Hope needs an object. Setting realistic goals jointly with a patient is one way of restoring and maintaining hope. This can be initiated by asking the patient, 'And what do you hope will come out of this consultation?'.

It may be necessary to break down an ultimate (probably unrealistic) goal into a series of (more realistic) mini-goals. Thus, if a patient says, 'I want to be cured' or a paraplegic says, 'I want to walk again', an initial reply could be:

> 'I hear what you are saying . . . but that, I suppose, is your ultimate goal. I think it might be helpful if we could agree on a series of more short term goals. Reaching these would give us all a sense of achievement. Does that seem sensible to you?'

Setting goals is an integral part of caring for patients with an incurable disease, including terminal cancer. In one study, doctors and nurses in palliative care units set significantly more goals than did their counterparts in a general hospital.[9]

Table 1.1 Factors that influence hope in the terminally ill

Decrease	Increase
Feeling devalued	Feeling valued
Abandonment and isolation 'conspiracy of silence' 'there is nothing more which can be done'	Meaningful relationship(s) reminiscence humour
Lack of direction/goals	Realistic goals
Unrelieved pain and discomfort	Pain and symptom relief

Hope is also related to other aspects of life and relationships (Table 1.1). Communication of painful truth does not equal destruction of hope (see p.17). Hope of recovery is replaced by an alternative hope.

In patients close to death, hope tends to become focused on

● being rather than achieving

● relationship with others

● relationship with God or a higher being.

It is possible for hope to increase when a person is close to death, provided care and comfort remain satisfactory.[10] When there is little else left to hope for, it is still realistic to hope

● not to be left alone to die

● for a peaceful death.

PART TWO

Psychosocial Aspects of Care

Communication · Breaking bad news
Strategies for coping with uncertainty
Psychological aspects of terminal illness
Care of the relatives · Spiritual care
Religious and cultural needs
Bereavement · Children and bereavement

Communication

'Communications, like tumours, may be benign or malignant. They may also be invasive, and the effects of bad communication with a patient may metastasize to the family. Truth is one of the most powerful therapeutic agents available to us, but we still need to develop a proper understanding of its clinical pharmacology and to recognize optimum timing and dosage in its use. Similarly, we need to understand the closely related metabolisms of hope and denial.'[11]

The aims of communication are to

- reduce uncertainty
- enhance relationships
- give the patient and family a direction in which to move.

The basic message a patient wants to hear at a time of increasing uncertainty is:

'No matter what happens to you, we will not desert you.' (acceptance)

'You may be dying, but you are still important to us.' (affirmation)

Only part of this can be said in words:

> 'We can relieve your pain and can ease most other symptoms.'
>
> 'I will see you regularly.'
>
> 'One of us will always be available.'
>
> 'Let's work out how best we can help you and your family.'

A large part of the message is conveyed to the patient by nonverbal means. Nonverbal communication includes

- facial expression
- eye contact
- posture, including whether sitting or standing
- pitch and pace of voice
- touch.

Touch is an important means of conveying re-assurance and comfort, e.g. holding a patient's hand – although cultural norms must be borne in mind.

Getting started

- make time for an unhurried conversation without interruption
- privacy is important
- introduce self by name and shake hands
- sit down to indicate you have time to listen
- make eye contact
- avoid medical jargon.

A patient-led agenda is particularly important in patients with many symptoms. A formal systematic enquiry alone may leave the doctor uncertain as to what to tackle first – and add to the patient's distress by failing to develop a clear plan of campaign. Useful ways of starting include:

> 'What do you hope will come out of this consultation?'
>
> 'Can you tell me about your problems?'
>
> 'How are you feeling?'

It is often helpful to allow a new patient to tell her story from the time the illness first manifested – even if this was several years ago, e.g. 'We have not met before. It would help me if you could start right from the beginning'. This often throws up unresolved concerns or resentments from the past which may be crucial to present management and support.

Active listening

- nod from time to time to show that you are still paying attention
- if the patient stops in the middle of a sentence, repeat her last three words; this gives permission to continue, and the offer is generally accepted
- pick up on cues, e.g. 'It's like Granny's illness' — 'What do you mean "It's like Granny's illness"?'
- keep the interview focused
- reflect questions back, e.g. 'What do *you* think the operation was for?'
- ask about feelings, e.g. 'How did/does that make you feel?'
- validate feelings, e.g. 'It's natural you should feel like that'
- watch body language and pick up on nonverbal cues
- summarize and check the accuracy of your understanding of the patient's problems
- if there is a long list of problems, ask the patient to prioritize them.

Asking questions

One of the primary aims of a consultation is to elicit the patient's feelings and concerns. Some questions tend to restrict the amount of information shared by the patient. Thus

- *leading questions* tend to produce the answer the questioner wants to hear, e.g. 'Are you feeling better today?'
- *closed questions* tend to produce the answer yes or no, e.g. 'Have you any pain?'
- *open questions* allow the patient to express feelings and concerns, e.g. 'How are you feeling today?' and 'How have you been coping since we last met?'

Without open questions, it is usually impossible to discover how the patient is really feeling, and find out what the main concerns are.

Avoid distancing

Distancing is behaviour by which caregivers avoid becoming involved with a patient on a psychosocial level, generally without being aware of it. Common ways by which doctors distance themselves include

- nonverbal messages:
  always busy
  general demeanour
  facial expression
  tone of voice

- placing people in diagnostic categories, e.g. 'She's a breast cancer' or 'He's a difficult patient'

- never enquiring beyond the physical, i.e. never asking, 'How are you coping?' or 'How are you feeling?'

- closed questions

- deflecting patient's questions

- paying selective attention to 'safe' physical aspects:
  Patient 'I am worried about myself. I am losing weight and the pain in my back has come back again'
  Doctor 'Tell me about the pain'

- premature normalization, e.g. by saying when a patient starts to cry, 'Don't worry, everyone in your position feels upset' instead of, 'I can see you're upset. Can you bear to tell me exactly what is upsetting you?'

- premature or false re-assurance, e.g. 'Don't worry. You leave it to me. Everything will be all right'

- using euphemisms to mislead

- jollying along/expecting the patient to keep up a brave face, e.g. 'Come on, the sun's shining; there's no need to look so glum!'

Breaking bad news

Bad news is information that drastically and unpleasantly alters a patient's view of her future. In practice, it is seldom a question of 'to tell or not to tell', but more a matter of 'when and how to tell'.

Breaking bad news generally causes distress to both the patient and the newsgiver. It is necessary to be prepared for a strong emotional reaction, e.g. tears, anger. Telling the patient and family together avoids difficulties and mistrust. It also gives opportunity for mutual support.

The principle 'never destroy hope' is sometimes used as a reason for not informing a patient of the seriousness of the situation. False optimism is a potent destroyer of hope. On the other hand, a total catharsis by the doctor of all that is negative either to the patient or to the family may irreversibly destroy hope and result in intractable anxiety and despair. It is necessary to apply two parallel principles, namely

● never lie to a patient

● avoid thoughtless candour.

Gradual communication of the truth within the context of continued support and encouragement almost always leads to enhancement of hope (see p.11).

The doctor – patient relationship is founded on trust.
It is fostered by honesty but poisoned by deceit.

The doctor's relationship with the patient should not be compromised by making unwise (and unethical) promises to the relatives about not informing the patient. It is necessary to check awareness, i.e. determine where the patient is at present in terms of knowledge and understanding, and to proceed according to her responses.

If a patient indicates directly or indirectly that she does not wish to regard her illness as fatal, it is wrong to force the truth on her. She is using denial as a coping strategy and, as such, it is vital to present wellbeing. Few patients adopt such a stance permanently.

Patients who want to know more about their condition often ask indirectly:

'And what's the next step, doctor?'

'How long do you reckon this will go on, doctor?'

'I'm not getting any better, am I?'

Sometimes a doctor needs to use open questions to find out if a patient wants more information:

'What things have been running through your mind as to the cause of your symptoms?'

'This illness is dragging on. Are there times when you find yourself looking on the black side?'

Alternatively, it may be helpful to ask the patient:

'Are you the sort of person who likes to know what's happening or do you like to leave it all to the doctor?'

If the patient indicates they prefer to 'leave it to the doctors', this should be accepted as the *present* position. Permission should be given, however, to ask questions at any time should the patient wish to.

If the patient wants more information

- give a 'warning shot' before stating the diagnosis, e.g. 'Tests indicate that we could be dealing with something serious'
- tailor the information to the patient's perceived needs
- use a hierarchy of euphemisms:
  some abnormal cells
  a kind of tumour
  a bit cancerous

- be prepared to stop if the patient indicates that she has heard enough, e.g. 'Well, I'll leave all that in your hands, doctor'
- explore how she *feels* about the situation.

Doctors generally underestimate what a patient already knows.

For most people, cancer is an emotive word. If asked directly 'Have I got cancer?', first discover what the patient understands by cancer. If to the patient it means an agonizing death, it is important before confirming the diagnosis to explain that this need not be because treatments are now available to relieve pain and other symptoms should they develop.

After giving bad news, try to offer some good news – but not before finding out how the patient feels about the bad news. Good news might include

- what can be done to relieve pain and other symptoms

- there will still be good times despite the progressive illness.

Truth has a broad spectrum with gentleness at one end and harshness at the other. Patients prefer gentle truth. As far as possible, soften the initial impact of emotionally negative words:

Not 'You've got cancer.'	*But* 'Tests indicate that it is a form of cancer.'
Not 'You've got 3 months to live.'	*But* 'Time is probably limited.'

Use words with positive rather than negative overtones:

Not 'You've got weaker.'	*But* 'Energy, at the moment, is limited.'
Not 'Things are getting worse.'	*But* 'Things don't seem to be so good this week.'

Euphemisms are legitimate if used to express truth gently; they are wrong if used to deceive.

Dealing with anger

Anger is a normal response to bad news and may be directed at the doctor. It is important not to become defensive. Instead, listen carefully to what is being expressed, clarify the causes and indicate that, 'Given what's been happening to you, I'm not surprised you feel so angry'. Judgements about the appropriateness of the focus of the anger are not helpful.

In summary

- get the physical surroundings right, e.g. privacy
- establish what the patient knows and what she wants to know
- use open questions
- the initial blow may be softened by stressing what medical science can offer, perhaps erring on the side of optimism

- do not give false hope

- do not be afraid of silence

- pay attention to reactions

- check back to ensure that the message has been taken in

- make sure you are answering the question being asked

- try to get the patient to come to her own conclusion

- do not give more information than is wanted

- accept denial but do not collude with it, e.g. 'Perhaps we'd better just wait and see'

- have the confidence to say, 'I don't know'

- allow expression of strong emotion, e.g. tears, anger

- acknowledge the awfulness of uncertainty and explore the problems it creates

- establish a positive direction in which to move

- not talking does not prevent the inevitable from happening

- be honest with yourself; when someone says he wants to protect the patient, he is often trying to protect himself.

Strategies for coping with uncertainty

Prognosis depends on many different factors – both physical and psychological. Although mean and median figures for survival are available, these relate to 'Mr Average' and not to the patient in your consultation room. When a patient asks about prognosis, try to avoid giving a specific length of time:

> *Patient* 'How long have I got, doctor?'

> *Doctor* 'I don't know – and nobody knows . . . there are just too many factors to take into account – both physical and psychological . . . I don't know.'

Many terminally ill patients die sooner than the doctor's estimate.[12] If given a specific time, some patients act as if the doctor's estimate is divine prophecy. In consequence, they become increasingly fearful as the deadline approaches and, indeed, may suffer some noncancerous catastrophe on the day of their predicted death – and die.

Having established that nobody knows, it is important to

- ask the patient what made him ask; this may unearth specific concerns which can then be discussed
- acknowledge that *living with uncertainty* can be very difficult, e.g. 'That's hard isn't it . . . having to live with the uncertainty'
- discuss coping strategies:
    a rolling horizon
    hope for the best but plan for the worst
    reaching anniversaries
    living one day at a time.

A rolling horizon

Here the anticipated survival is 4–6 months or more:

'Given how you are now, you should work on the basis that you will be well enough to do what you want to do for the next two/three months. So go home and fill your diary out for this period of time – with the high expectation that you will be able to fulfil your commitments. If in 4 weeks time, you are still as good as you are now or better, then fill your diary out for another month, and so on.'

Hope for the best but plan for the worst

Here the anticipated survival is 2–3 months, possibly more:

'Given how things have been and are now, it is difficult to plan confidently for the future. What I suggest is that you adopt a "cross-eyed" approach. With one eye plan as if things are going to work out fairly well and, with the other, make alternative plans in case things work out not so well . . . How does that seem to you?'

Reaching anniversaries

Here the outlook seems very poor, but the patient is still hoping for some time. In this circumstance, it may help to identify anniversaries or special events which will occur in the next few months, and suggest to the patient that she should aim to reach them one by one.

Living one day at a time

Some people do this successfully for months, but it can lead to wasted time and opportunities because the patient sets no medium term goals. However, in people who are within a few weeks of death, it is often a helpful strategy. An alternative is to suggest living one or two weeks at a time.

Beware the tendency of some patients to 'extremize':

> *Doctor* 'It could be 2–3 months, or it could be 2–3 years.'

> *Patient* (later to family) 'The doctor said I had only 2 months to live.' *or* 'The doctor said I had at least 5 years.'

When pressed for more information, remember

- if deteriorating *month by month*, the prognosis is likely to be *months*

- if deteriorating *week by week*, the prognosis is likely to be *weeks*

- If deteriorating *day by day*, the prognosis is likely to be *days*.

But how long is *months, weeks, days* ?

Psychological aspects of terminal illness

Responses to loss

Similar psychological responses occur in various circumstances, ranging from loss of a job, amputation, divorce or bereavement to the anticipated loss of one's own life. They include

- shock

- emotional numbness

- denial

- anger

- anxiety

- guilt

- grief

- resignation or acceptance.

These responses do not necessarily occur in sequence. Several may occur together and some may not occur at all. In cancer patients, more marked responses may be seen

- at or shortly after the time of diagnosis
- at the time of the first recurrence
- at each major sign of disease progression.

There is no one right way of responding and adjusting to a poor prognosis. The doctor's task is to help the patient adjust in the best way possible, given that particular patient's background – familial, cultural and spiritual. Many people have a combination of inner resources and good support from the family and others which enable them to cope without prolonged and disabling distress.

Psychological problems

Many palliative care patients experience significant psychological problems. About 10% have an identifiable psychiatric disorder. Problems are also common among patients' relatives.

Denial

Denial is a common coping mechanism in the dying. It signifies an ability to obliterate or minimize threatening reality by ignoring it. It may be associated with physiological and other nonverbal evidence of anxiety. Most patients continue to make use of denial to a varying extent. Patients experience conflict between the wish to know the truth and the wish to avoid anxiety. Denial is one way of coping with this. Professional intervention may be needed when denial persists and interferes with

- the acceptance of treatment
- planning for the future
- relationships.

Anger

Anger may be an appropriate short term reaction to the diagnosis of serious illness, but persistent anger is a problem. If displaced on to the family or staff, it tends to alienate those who want to care. Anger can also interfere with the acceptance of limitations, and may stop a patient from making positive adjustments to physical disability.

Anxiety

Anxiety often relates to uncertainty and fear of the future, and the threat of separation from loved ones. It may present with physical symptoms such as nausea or diarrhoea, rather than with psychological complaints. Many cancer patients sleep badly, have frightening dreams or are reluctant to be left alone at night. Explanation about the illness and special techniques such as relaxation training and cognitive-behavioural therapy are helpful forms of management but some patients also need anxiolytic drugs. If depressive symptoms are present as well, a sedative antidepressant drug should be used.

Depression

Recognizing depression is important because patients often have a good response to antidepressant drugs. Depression is often missed because symptoms overlap with appropriate grief about dying (sadness) and with the somatic symptoms of cancer, i.e. anorexia, constipation, weight loss. Many patients also try to hide their negative feelings. Pointers to depression include

- persistent low mood (but diurnal variation)
- loss of interest and inability to feel pleasure
- feelings of guilt or unworthiness
- hopelessness/despair
- physical manifestations of anxiety (sweating, tremor, panic attacks)
- suicide attempts/persistent thoughts about suicide
- requests for euthanasia.

Paranoid states

Paranoid states may be caused by corticosteroids, biochemical disturbance, cerebral metastases or psychological factors. For example, unable to accept that he is dying, the patient believes there is a plot to kill him or the treatment is the cause of his deterioration.

Communication problems

Staff may not give as much information as patients and families need, even when asked directly. Within families, there is a conflict between the wish to confide and to receive emotional and practical support, and the wish to protect others from distress, particularly children or frail parents. A conspiracy of silence is a source of tension. It blocks discussion of the future and preparation for parting. If it is not resolved, the bereaved often experience much regret.

Other problems

Cancer related   e.g. impact on sexual function; difficulty in accepting a colostomy, paraplegia or the effects of cerebral secondaries.

Cancer always changes family psychodynamics, either for better or worse.

Treatment related   e.g. adverse drug effects such as hair loss.

Patients may want to share in decisions about when to stop treatment aimed at prolonging life. Fear of death may make some want to go on even when adverse effects are severe and the chance of improvement is minimal. Others may wish to opt for a shorter life of better quality when doctors are advocating more aggressive measures.

Concurrent   e.g. a bereavement or a pre-existing psychiatric illness.

Management

Psychological problems are easily overlooked by doctors and nurses. Open questions, e.g. 'How are you feeling?' and 'How are you coping?' may facilitate the expression of negative emotion. Suspicion that there is marked anxiety or severe depression may be confirmed by asking the patient to complete a screening test such as the Hospital Anxiety and Depression (HAD) Scale.

Some psychological problems could be prevented by

- good staff – patient communication, giving information according to individual need
- good staff – patient relationships, with continuity of care
- enabling patients to have some control over the management of their illness.

Anxiolytics and/or antidepressants are often necessary adjuncts to psychological and social measures. Appropriate treatment will enable the patient to

- have a better quality of life during the illness
- prepare for death
- retain individuality and self-respect to the end.

Care of the relatives

The care of the family is an integral part of the care of the dying. A contented family increases the likelihood of a contented patient. Relative – doctor communication generally needs to be initiated and maintained by the doctor. It is easy to neglect the family because they are reluctant to trouble the doctor 'because he's so busy'.

Telling the relatives

For the family and patient to be too far out of step in relation to knowledge about the diagnosis and the prognosis can create a barrier between them. A common initial reaction is 'You won't tell him, will you, doctor?' or 'We'd prefer you not to tell him, doctor'. This should be seen as an initial shock reaction, stemming from the relative's own instinctive fear of death coupled with a desire to protect a loved one from hurt. It should not be used as an excuse for saying nothing to the patient.

If the family and patient are to be mutually supportive it is necessary to help the relatives move forward from this initial reaction to a position of greater openness and trust. *The family cannot forbid the doctor from discussing diagnosis and prognosis with the patient.* Indeed, given the ethic of medical confidentiality, it is clear that relatives can be told only with the implicit or explicit permission of the patient, and not the other way round.

In practice, there is much to be said for joint interviews at the time of diagnosis and later – patient, relative, doctor and nurse. This prevents collusion and a conspiracy of silence by which the patient is excluded from the process of information sharing. In addition, the presence of a nurse facilitates subsequent clarification of what the doctor said.

The doctor should also make an opportunity to see both the patient and the close family apart from each other. Further separate or joint interviews can then be arranged as necessary. As with the patient, it is generally not necessary or wise initially to tell the family the whole truth (as you perceive it) at one time. The relatives also need time to adjust to the implications of the diagnosis.

Involvement in inpatient care

Admission to hospital or a palliative care unit may be seen as a defeat by the family. It helps if the doctor emphasizes that he is surprised that they have managed to cope for so long and that now, with the need for 24-hour care, it is impossible for them to continue without a break. It should be emphasized that the presence of relatives and close friends is regarded as important for the patient's continued wellbeing. If practical, unrestricted visits should be encouraged.

The relatives' separation anxiety may be reduced by encouraging them to help in the care of the patient, e.g. adjusting pillows, refilling a water jug, helping with a blanket bath, assisting at meals if necessary. Some relatives need to be taught how to visit, to behave as they would at home, e.g. sit and read a book or newspaper, knit, watch the television together. It may need to be emphasized that it is not necessary to keep up a tiring patter of conversation.

Overnight accommodation should be arranged when necessary, possibly using a divan in the patient's room or guest accommodation if available and convenient.

Planning for discharge

A proportion of patients with terminal illness, particularly cancer, improve following admission as a result of pain and symptom management. They become physically independent and no longer need to be inpatients.

Many relatives have fears about what will happen should the patient be discharged. A daytime visit or a weekend at home often does much to allay their fear – or confirms after all that discharge is impractical. A doctor (as well as other team members) should discuss matters with the relatives both before and after a trial period at home. Future plans can then be made on the basis of comments by both the family and the patient.

Patients are sometimes overprotected by their family. For example, even though still capable of driving, visiting the pub or betting shop, they are not allowed to do so. It is necessary in these cases to help the relatives to accept the patient's need (and right) to maintain the maximum possible degree of independence. An explanation that a sudden dramatic deterioration is unlikely will help ease the family's apprehension. They also need clear guidance about what to do in an emergency, i.e. whether to call the general practitioner or the hospital/palliative care unit.

Explanation of treatment

Terminally, it is advisable to tell the relatives that, because the patient is less well and swallowing is difficult, medicine may need to be given by injection to prevent pain or other distress recurring. If pneumonia develops, the doctor should explain that he plans to treat it symptomatically and not use antibiotics.

After the patient's death

Because bereavement has both a morbidity and a mortality, palliative care does not end when the patient dies. Many relatives have false feelings of guilt:

'If only I'd done this!'

'Do you think, if he'd gone to the hospital sooner, he wouldn't have died?'

Opportunity should be given for such feelings to be aired and questions raised.

Spiritual care

'*Palliative care integrates psychological, social and spiritual aspects of care so that patients may come to terms with their own death as fully and constructively as they can.*'

Spiritual relates to values (ultimate issues and life principles) and to a person's search for meaning and purpose in life. It also refers to experiences and relationships which transcend sensory phenomena.

Religion is a shared framework of theistic beliefs and rituals which give expression to spiritual concerns.

The spiritual dimension may also be viewed as the integrating component, holding together physical, psychological and social dimensions (Figure 2.1).

For those nearing the end of life, there is commonly an increased or renewed need for

● affirmation and acceptance

● forgiveness and reconciliation

● the discovery of meaning and direction.

Death is not the ultimate tragedy of life. The ultimate tragedy is depersonalization, e.g.

● dying in an alien and sterile area

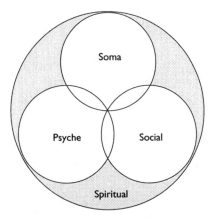

Figure 2.1   Total care for a person involves four dimensions.

● separation from the spiritual nourishment of a fellow human being

● hopelessness and despair.

Glimpses of spirituality at Sobell House[13]
In talking together at Sobell House about spirituality, a rich mixture of experiences, insights and feelings has emerged which defies simple definition. There is both meaning and mystery, a sense of interconnectedness and relationship alongside an awareness of our individuality.

We may connect with the spiritual dimension through the beauty of the natural world, through our relationships with others, through religious practices, through painting or music, or other forms of art. But there is also a sense of awe and aloneness on this journey. We may have faith, and we may search and question. Our feelings may shift from courage and hope to fear – and back again. There may be joy, love, forgiveness and truth, as well as pain and suffering. Through all, a dynamic energy takes us along our different paths. It is an area of experience where we may have more to learn from patients and relatives than we have to teach, more to receive than to give.

Whether apparent or not, most patients are in need of spiritual help and are seeking answers:[14]

Meaning of suffering and pain Why do I have to suffer? Why has this happened to me?

Value systems What value is there in money, material possessions, and social position? What is valuable in my life?

Quest after God Is there a God? Why does God allow me to suffer like this?

The meaning of life What is the meaning of life in a time of serious illness? What's the point of it all? What is my relationship with God?

Guilt feelings I have done many wrong things. How can they be corrected? How can I be forgiven?

Life after death Is there life after death? How can I believe in life after death? What is it like?

Although relatively few patients discuss the spiritual aspects of life and death with their doctor, the majority do so with another team member or with relatives and close friends. It is important to be aware that the dying do consider such issues, and to be able to respond sympathetically if a patient chooses to raise them. Patients are very perceptive and they are unlikely to embarrass a doctor if they sense that communication at this level will cause discomfort.

A doctor's primary responsibility is to help maintain an environment which is supportive of the patient. This includes the relief of symptoms so that the patient is able to reflect on life and its meaning. It is important not to fall into the trap of thinking that you understand the spiritual pain the patient is suffering. Further, it is not generally helpful if a doctor tries to provide neat answers to a patient's questions. Ultimately, each one has to find answers which are personally satisfying. Sharing in not knowing is more comforting than being left feeling other people have all the answers.

When appropriate, the doctor should alert the chaplain/priest/rabbi to the fact that 'Mr Brown is seriously ill and may appreciate a visit'. Respect for the patient as a person does not allow the imposition on him of one's own faith (or lack of it). Many patients are comforted by the discovery that their doctor has a religious faith.

Some possible indicators of spiritual need, pain or dis-ease[15]

- a sense of hopelessness, meaninglessness, powerlessness, e.g. 'I'd be better off dead than living like this'. Such a patient may become withdrawn and suicidal

- intense suffering, e.g. 'I can't endure this any more' and 'What's the point of going on like this?' Includes loneliness, isolation, vulnerability. Challenges the care being given, e.g. 'If this is the best you can do, I'd rather be dead'

- remoteness of God, inability to trust, break with religious and cultural ties, e.g. 'I don't believe in God any more', 'I can't ask him for help' and 'How can I trust people if even God has let me down?'

- anger towards God, religion, clergy, e.g. 'Why? Why me?' and 'What have I done to deserve this?'

- undue stoicism and desire to show others how to do it, e.g. 'I must not let God/my church/my family down'

- a sense of guilt or shame, i.e. illness means punishment; bitter and unforgiving of self/others, e.g. 'I don't deserve to get better'

- concern with moral/ethical nature of treatment. Feelings of unworthiness may relate to guilt and shame, e.g. 'Do you think I should have this treatment/operation? I've had my life'

- unresolved feelings about death manifesting as fear of sleep and the dark, i.e. the longer you stay awake the longer you put off death. Any illness may concentrate the mind and raise questions of what is beyond death, e.g. 'Letting go into what?'

Evaluation

Nonverbal behaviour

- observe affect, e.g. does the person's affect or attitude convey loneliness, depression, anger, agitation or anxiety?

- observe behaviours, e.g. does the person pray and/or does he make use of religious reading material?

Verbal behaviour

- does the person seem to complain out of proportion to his illness?

- are there reports of sleeping difficulties?

- are abnormally high doses of sedation or pain medication needed?

- does the person refer to God in any way?

- does the person talk about:
  prayer, faith, hope or anything of a religious nature?
  church functions which are part of his life?

- does the person express concern about the meaning of life?

Environment

- does the person have visitors from church? Are they supportive or do they seem to leave the person feeling upset?

- does the person have with him:
    religious reading material?
    religious medals or other religious objects?

- has the person received religious get well cards?

- does the person use religious pictures, artwork or music to keep his spirits up?

Religious and cultural needs

(John Barton)

'**Respect for privacy, dignity and religious and cultural beliefs**. The [Patient's] Charter Standard is that all health services should make provision so that proper personal consideration is shown to you, for example by ensuring that your privacy, dignity and religious and cultural beliefs are respected.'[16]

For many people, religion is an important element in their lives, from which they derive inspiration and strength.

Every society develops a set of arrangements to enable members to live peacefully with each other. These arrangements form part of that society's culture. Thus, a culture may be defined as the way of living adopted by a specific group of people.

It is important to reach an understanding with each patient and her relatives about religious and cultural needs. People should be cared for where they are in their beliefs and not where we happen to be.

Christianity

Belief in God revealed in Jesus Christ and at work in people and events in the world today through the Holy Spirit. The Church is the worshipping community of believers. God's grace and strength is given in many ways, particularly through the Bible, prayers and sacraments.

Most hospitals have a chapel and many patients value its peace and quiet, e.g. 'I feel a lot better after sitting here in the chapel'.

Three chaplains are appointed in most hospitals:

Church of England (Anglican)
Roman Catholic
Free Church – includes Methodist, Baptist, United Reformed, Congregational, Salvation Army, Moravian, Brethren, Society of Friends (Quakers), Pentecostal, Seventh Day Adventist.

Adherents of certain sects, e.g. Christian Scientists, Jehovah's Witnesses and Mormons, may be reluctant to be seen by a hospital chaplain.

Judaism

Belief in one universal God who is to be worshipped. The Jewish Sabbath is from Friday evening until Saturday evening. There are a number of important Jewish Festivals during the year:

Pesach (first day of Passover – April)
Shavuot (Feast of Weeks – May)
Rosh Hashanah (Jewish New Year – September)
Yom Kippur (Day of Atonement – September)
Succoth (first day of the Feast of Tabernacles – October).

Orthodox Jews eat meat only when it has been killed by their own trained people (Kosher). They never eat pork. Some hospitals store deep-frozen Kosher meals.

The local Jewish community generally organizes a group of people to care for patients in hospital. Most families want to be present at the moment of death. Some members of the family or the community may wish to remain in the hospital with the body after death.

After death, it is advisable to wear disposable gloves so that there is no direct contact with the body. Members of the Jewish community will probably wash and prepare the body for burial. No mutilation of the body is allowed unless an autopsy is required for legal reasons. The funeral is generally held within 24 h.

Relatives are encouraged to express their grief openly – 3 days of intense grief, followed by grieving periods of 7 days and 30 days for re-adjustment. The Jewish community is very supportive during this time.

Islam

Islam is the Arabic word for submission, surrender, obedience. 'There is no God but Allah.' Mohammed is the prophet sent by God. Muslims come from all over the world. In the UK, most are from India, Bangladesh, Pakistan, North Africa and Arab countries.

The *Qur'an* is the Holy Book revealed to the prophet Mohammed. The five pillars of Islam are

- there is only one God
- prayers five times a day
- almsgiving
- fasting
- pilgrimage to Mecca.

Islam does not have an organized ministry comparable to the Christian clergy. There is respect for holy men (imams), which could include hospital chaplains. Friday is the Holy Day.

Other features include

- diet – pork and alcohol are forbidden, some are vegetarian
- modesty – the women are reluctant to undress for examination
- cleanliness – great importance attached to personal hygiene
- prayer – facing Mecca, i.e. south-east.

When dying, friends may read from the *Qur'an* and whisper the Muslim articles of faith in order to bring peace to the soul.[17]

The body should not be touched by the hospital staff. Disposable gloves should be used for the Last Offices. The head should be turned to the right before rigor mortis sets in. Family members of the same sex as the deceased may attend to the washing of the body. The body is buried as quickly as possible. Autopsy is allowed only if legally necessary. Cremation is prohibited; coffins are not used.

Many Asian people with their close-knit families find it difficult to accept our Western idea of restricted visiting. The whole family feel bound to visit as often as possible.

Hinduism

Hinduism dates back to about 2500 BC. There is no single prophet, no formal creed or central authority.

Worship is often in the home. Even in a temple there is no set pattern of worship. There is a complex system of gods and goddesses who are subsidiary to the Supreme Being. The guru (teacher, guide) occupies an important place in guiding the Hindu on his path through life.

Beliefs include transmigration of the soul with an indefinite number of re-incarnations until the attainment of Nirvana or fusion with the Supreme Being.

Other features include

- names – personal name, complementary name, and family name
- diet – the cow is sacred and Hindus are forbidden to eat beef. Many Hindus are vegetarian
- modesty – many Asian women find undressing embarrassing
- cleanliness – prefer to wash in running water. The left hand is used for unclean tasks, e.g. toilet; the right hand for clean tasks, e.g. eating.

When a Hindu is dying, a Hindu priest should be contacted if the family wish it. Relatives often go home and do not stay at the bedside.[18]

A Hindu prefers to die at home, preferably on the floor near Mother Earth. He may want to do this in hospital. The relatives should be asked about washing the body etc. They may want to do this and put on new clothes. Autopsy is not forbidden but is considered distasteful. Cremation is usual.

Sikhism

Founded in the fifteenth century AD, Sikhism is a society in which every member works for the common good. Sikh means disciple. Most come from the Punjab.

Sikhism teaches that everyone should have direct communication with God, and that none should have special privileges by reason of birth, wealth, religion, race or sex. The way of salvation is through a good life of kindness to others and concern for family and society. Sikhs believe in re-incarnation.

Women have equal status with men and are outgoing and ready to enter society. There are no priests.

A Sikh is identified by five marks, the removal of any of which would be distressing and offensive

- uncut hair and beard
- comb ('top knot' of hair) and turban
- steel bangle – reminder of the unity of God
- sword – now often worn as a brooch
- shorts – reminder of sexual discipline.

Other features include

- names – personal name, title Singh (lion) for men and Kaur (princess) for women, and family name
- diet – beef is prohibited
- modesty – women prefer to be examined by a female doctor or to have a female chaperone
- prayers – privacy for personal prayers is appreciated.

When close to death the relevant part of the Sikh scriptures are read. Sikh hymns are read over the dead body in the home. There is no objection to staff handling the body. Cremation is favoured; ashes are thrown into water.

Buddhism

Buddhism arose against a background of Hinduism in the sixth century BC. Buddha is not revered as a god, but as an example of a way of life. Buddhahood must be realized within ourselves through prayer and virtuous conduct.

Buddhists believe in re-incarnation. They accept responsibility for their lives because the consequences of present actions will have an effect on future lives, until Nirvana is attained where individuals lose identity and merge with the Supreme Being. Buddhists may appreciate a time of peace and quiet for meditation to help achieve inner calm. Buddhism condemns contraception, abortion and euthanasia. It accepts blood transfusion and transplants. No foods are forbidden but some Buddhists are vegetarian.

Helping people is fundamental to the Buddhist ideal and the patient will always respect those (doctor, nurse etc.) helping him. The family should be consulted whenever possible about specific wishes or needs. It may be possible to contact a local Buddhist priest when a Buddhist patient is dying.

A dying Buddhist may wish to maintain clarity of thought as long as possible and may decline analgesics if these induce drowsiness.[19] There are no specific rituals related to Last Offices; anyone may prepare the body. Cremation is usual. White is the colour of mourning.

Bereavement

(Marilyn Relf)

> '"Mourning [grieving] is not forgetting" he said gently, his helplessness vanishing and his voice becoming wise. "It is an undoing. Every minute tie has to be untied and something permanent and valuable recovered and assimilated from the knot. The end is gain, of course. Blessed are they that mourn [grieve], for they shall be made strong. But the process is like all other human births, painful and long and dangerous."'[20]
>
> 'An affliction of the heart may be physical as well as spiritual. Always it is the whole person who must be healed. For what hurts one part hurts the whole.'[21]

People often think of grief as an emotional experience. It is – but it is also a physical, intellectual, social and spiritual experience.[22] Grief not only affects how a person feels, it also affects behaviour. Some of the many and varied reactions are listed below (Table 2.1). Note how grief may lead to apathy in some but overactivity in others – or both in the same person at different times.

The process of grief

Personal crises

- provide new insights
- change one's understanding of the world
- have a major formative impact.

Table 2.1   Common reactions to grief

Physical reactions

Sighing	Weakness and fatigue
Tachycardia	Increased blood pressure
Muscular tension	Sleep disturbances
Decreased resistance to illness	Weight and appetite change
Self-neglect	Increased sensory awareness

Emotional reactions

Numbness	Guilt
Sadness	Anger
Helplessness	Bitterness
Hopelessness	Vengefulness
Despair	Relief
Feeling of being lost	Spiritual connectedness
Confusion	Peacefulness
Yearning	Euphoria

Behavioural reactions

Searching	Decreased activity/apathetic
Disorientation	Detached from surroundings
Poor concentration	Withdrawn from friends and activities
Blaming others	
Pre-occupied	Forgetful
Seeking solitude	Crying
	Increased activity

Bereavement is the greatest personal crisis which many people ever have to face. Grief is a transitional process.[23] By grieving, the bereaved person adjusts to the loss and the meaning of that loss in her life. In other words, the reality of an external event is assimilated internally.

In the UK, changes in society over the last 50 years have affected the way loss and bereavement are perceived

● people expect to live longer and be healthier because of improved health care, e.g. antibiotics, better nutrition and the absence of war

● people commonly do not experience bereavement before adulthood because of decreased infant and child mortality

● families are smaller and more scattered

● people live in smaller units.

The bereaved, particularly the elderly, feel more isolated and turn to professionals (notably the general practitioner) or to support groups (such as Cruse) for help and understanding. Many people do not easily seek help. This increases their feeling of isolation.

The process of grief has been described in several different models

- phases of grief[23]
- tasks of mourning[24]
- dimensions of loss[25]
- dual process.[26]

Understanding these models of grief helps one to understand the impact of bereavement on an individual.

Phases of grief

Shock, numbness and disbelief

Initially, bereaved people may feel as if they are detached from reality. Because the reality of the death has not yet fully penetrated awareness, they may appear outwardly to have accepted the loss.

Separation and pain

'The absence of the dead person is everywhere palpable. The home and family environs seem full of painful reminders. Grief breaks over the bereaved in waves of distress. There is intense yearning, as if the dead person has been torn out of his body.'[23]

Shock and numbness gradually give way to intense feelings.

Searching behaviour is common

- 'seeing' the dead person in the street
- other misinterpretations, including hallucinations
- dreaming about the deceased
- revisiting favourite places hoping that the deceased might be there.

Despair

Despair sets in when it is realized that the lost person will not return. Poor concentration, anger, guilt, irritability, anxiety, restlessness and extreme sadness become common.

Acceptance

Bereaved people may be intellectually aware of the finality of the loss long before their emotions let them accept the truth. Depression and emotional swings may continue for more than a year after bereavement. Despair gradually gives way to acceptance of the loss.

Resolution and re-organization

As old patterns of life are given up, new patterns without the dead person are adopted and the bereaved person enters the phase of resolution or re-organization. Eventually the bereaved person is able to remember the deceased without being overwhelmed by sadness or other emotions and is ready to re-invest in the world.

This model implies a certain passivity. It is limited because it suggests that bereavement proceeds from one clearly identifiable reaction to another in an orderly fashion. This is not the case. The model should be used with care to avoid inappropriate behaviour towards bereaved people, such as hasty judgements of where individuals are or ought to be in their grief.

Tasks of mourning

The process of grief has also been described as a series of tasks to be completed by the bereaved in order to move towards resolution, i.e.

- accept the reality of the loss
- experience the pain of grief
- adjust to an environment in which the dead person is missing
- withdraw emotional energy and re-invest in other relationships and activities.

By encouraging the bereaved to work through the tasks of mourning, it is possible to facilitate the process of grief. The thought that something can be done and there is an end point is a powerful antidote to the feelings of helplessness experienced by most bereaved persons.

Dimensions of loss

This model focuses on how loss affects all the dimensions of life. It emphasizes that loss demands many adjustments, some of which are likely to be easier than others.

Identity

- how far has a person been able to accept the loss:
    intellectually?
    emotionally?

- how has it changed the person's concept of themselves and how has it affected self-esteem?

Emotional

- how freely is the person able to express emotions?

- how much has the person's emotional equilibrium been affected?

Spiritual

- what meaning has the bereaved ascribed to the experience?

- how has it affected religious beliefs, personal philosophy and the inner spiritual core?

Practical

- is the person able to deal with the day-to-day practicalities of life such as cooking, shopping, looking after himself and the home?

Physical

- how has the bereaved person's health been affected:
    having trouble sleeping?
    losing weight?
    experiencing stress-related symptoms?

Lifestyle

- has the bereaved person's lifestyle had to change?

- will she have to move house, start work, deal with finances?

Family and community

- how has the person's role changed:
    within the family, e.g. by taking on the deceased person's role as a mother or father?
    within society, e.g. being a widow rather than a wife?

- do friends treat the bereaved person differently?

- how isolated is the bereaved person?

Dual process

Most people cope after bereavement by oscillating between confronting grief (e.g. by going over the details of the experience and expressing their feelings) and avoiding grief (e.g. by avoiding memories, distracting themselves and keeping busy with other things). These are described as loss-oriented and restoration-oriented behaviour.

Loss-oriented behaviour focuses on the loss and the emotional reactions to it, whereas restoration-oriented behaviour encompasses a degree of suppression, distraction and 'taking time off' from grief. This enables people to carry on with their lives and attend to tasks previously undertaken by the deceased. As daily living is full of reminders of all that has been lost, people *oscillate* between the two ways of coping.

Bereaved people are more likely to manifest loss-oriented behaviour in the early months of bereavement but, in order to cope with daily life, some restoration-oriented behaviour is necessary. Thus a person may appear to be coping well one day and full of grief the next. Difficulties may emerge if the balance of behaviour is oriented exclusively on loss (chronic grief) or on restoration (absent grief).

Sources of help

In addition to the clergy, general practitioner, district nurse and social worker, there are two main organizations in the UK which offer help in bereavement or give advice.

Cruse
126 Sheen Road, Richmond, Surrey TW9 1UR
Tel: 0181 940 4818/9047

Cruse offers support to all bereaved people, both counselling and social activities. It has about 200 branches in the UK.

National Association of Bereavement Services
20 Norton Folgate, London E1 6DB
Tel: 0171 247 1080/0617

This is an umbrella organization for local bereavement services. It publishes a national directory of bereavement services.

Risk assessment in bereavement

'Statistical studies confirm that secure people whose experience of life has led to a reasonable trust in themselves and others will cope well with anticipated bereavements, provided they are well supported by a family who respects their need to grieve. However, multiple or unexpected and untimely losses of people on whom one depends or who depended on the survivor can overwhelm the most secure person, and lack of security and support can undermine a person's capacity to cope.'[27]

People vary in their response to bereavement. Grief may be

- immediate or delayed
- brief or seem unending
- severe or mild.

Most people work through their grief with the help of family and friends. Some report that they feel stronger and more mature. A significant minority suffer prolonged impairment of their physical and psychological health. Bereavement is associated with health risks. It

- predisposes people to physical and mental illness
- precipitates illness and death
- exacerbates existing illness
- leads to or exacerbates health threatening behaviour such as smoking, drinking and drug use

- results in an increased use of health services
- may lead to depression.[28]

Several factors are associated with a good or poor outcome. These can be identified at the time of bereavement and can be used to focus resources in order to prevent or ameliorate complicated grief.[27]

Mode of death

- was it timely or untimely?
- was it expected or unexpected?
- was it unduly disturbing for the relatives or key carers?

Deaths that are untimely, unexpected and/or unduly disturbing are likely to cause more severe and more prolonged grief. *The death of someone with terminal illness can still be unexpected.*

Nature of the relationship

How ambivalent was the relationship between the key carer and the patient? In a highly ambivalent relationship there is likely to be a more difficult bereavement. Often this manifests as persistent guilt feelings.

How necessary was the deceased for the key carer's sense of wellbeing, self-esteem or security? The more dependent the relationship the more all pervading the sense of loss.

Perceived support

- is the bereaved person able to share her feelings with family and friends?
- does she feel supported or isolated in her loss?

Anticipatory grieving

- were the family and patient able to talk about the illness, share feelings, and make plans for the future before the patient died?

Periods of denial by both patient and family are normal during a terminal illness but an excessive use of denial may make it harder for the survivor to start sharing with others after the patient's death.

Anger also may impede the process of grief. Angry people may deflect support and find themselves isolated.

Concurrent life events

● how much stress is the key carer/family currently facing?
  finances
  menopause
  children leaving home
  unemployment
  retirement

● how many people are dependent on the key carer, e.g. children or elderly relatives?

● has she time and space to grieve?

Previous losses

● how has the person grieved in the past?

● will the new loss uncover unresolved loss?

Medical history

● has the person a concurrent physical or psychological illness which is likely to be exacerbated by the loss?

● is there a history of alcoholism, drug abuse or suicidal behaviour?

The most positive factor in favour of a good outcome is a supportive family/friend who allows the bereaved person to express grief and to talk unconditionally about feelings for as long as is needed.[29]

Children and bereavement

(Ann Couldrick, Rosalyn Staveley)

More than 1% of children under 16 in the UK have lost at least one parent by death. The father comprises 80% of these parental deaths.[30]

Studies suggest that children are most deeply affected not by the actual loss but by

- the adverse changes in social and financial situation
- the significance of the relationship with the remaining parent
- the emotional climate in which the child is helped to come to terms with the loss.

There are several severe disruptions and changes which may affect the child

- the bereaved spouse is grieving
- other adults may or may not take on the dead parent's function
- the child may not understand what has happened because he has not been given clear information
- there may be changes of home and of school
- the family may have fewer social contacts
- there may be social and economic decline particularly when the father dies
- the surviving parent may remarry before the child has fully understood the dead parent is not going to return
- the child may be taken into care.

The majority of bereaved children do adjust normally, though they may show disturbance in behaviour at a much later date.

Adults frequently do not know what to expect and may deny that a child is affected. They are often unable to perceive or respond to the very clear signals of the child's distress. This is related to the adult's own way of dealing with the loss, which may be pathological.

The effect of bereavement on children

Physical responses

- sleep disturbances, i.e. insomnia and bad dreams, or retreating into sleep as an escape
- eating disorders, e.g. loss of appetite, compulsive eating, craving certain foods
- toileting difficulties, e.g. children previously continent who start to wet and soil are signalling distress

- physical symptoms may occur, e.g. rashes, fever, nausea, or existing conditions exacerbated, e.g. asthma, eczema. In an older child, symptoms frequently mimic those of the person who has died.

Emotional responses

- increased generalized anxiety often resulting in the child not wanting to leave home or go to school
- becoming more clinging and dependent
- exaggerated separation responses, e.g. intense distress when the carer walks out of the room or leaves for short periods
- rapid mood swings from euphoric and all right to weeping, depression, rejection of carer(s), withdrawal, or inappropriately aggressive responses in various situations.

Cognitive effects

- poor concentration
- loss of short term and/or long term memory
- poor or changed motivation, e.g. 'What is the point of anything now?'
- learning difficulties, e.g. an existing undiagnosed problem may become evident or a new difficulty may develop, the nature of which will depend upon the child's developmental stage.

Behavioural responses

- an obvious anxiety about or dislike of change in routine(s)
- regression to infant needs, e.g. wanting to be fed, rocked in parent's arms
- acting out behaviour reflecting an unconscious and often aggressive response which seems unrelated to feelings and needs, e.g. playing very loud music, dangerous competitive activities such as racing bikes or cars, and stealing
- putting on a brave face for the sake of the surviving parent, or because of a fear of losing control.

Approach the parent as a colleague

Remember, parents have expert knowledge about their children. Boost confidence and increase their feelings of competence by

- explaining the physical, emotional, cognitive and behavioural changes which might occur and re-assure parents that these are normal reactions for children

- recommending appropriate books and leaflets. These help some parents to gain intellectual mastery over the situation. Books to read with children can be important as a less direct way of approaching a discussion

- suggesting that parents encourage children to draw, paint or write about their experience of the loss and to talk about the implications if they wish

- suggesting that the children are encouraged to make a scrapbook of memories, e.g. photos, cards, letters, and collecting mementos and talking about these

- warning parents that children's play and interests may appear to revolve around dying, death and funerals. This is a natural way for children to work through their difficulties and gain a greater understanding of the world

- telling parents not to be too hard on themselves. It is normal sometimes to shout or be impatient with children – parents need only to be 'good enough'

- encouraging parents to be open with the children about how they are feeling themselves. In doing this, parents are modelling the honest expression of feelings:
  'I'm crying because I am sad'
  'I'm angry because we cannot do that together again'
  'I'm laughing because I am remembering how funny it was when . . .'

- encouraging parents to involve others (relatives, friends, teachers) for both practical help and emotional support

- being aware of and sensitive to the family belief and value systems – go along with their beliefs and values and do not impose your own – avoid 'ought' and 'should'

- encouraging parents to look after their own physical, practical and emotional needs. If they do, parents will be better able to deal with the children's needs and demands.

PART THREE

Symptom Management I

General principles · Pain
Pain in advanced cancer
Pain management · Nonopioids
Weak opioids · Strong opioids
Neuropathic pain · Useful definitions

General principles

The scientific approach to pain and symptom management can be summarized as

- evaluation
- explanation
- individualized treatment
- supervision
- attention to detail.

Patients are often reluctant to bother their doctor about minor symptoms such as dry mouth, altered taste, anorexia, pruritus, cough and insomnia. Enquiries should be made from time to time rather than rely on spontaneous reports.

Evaluation

Evaluation must precede treatment

The cancer itself is not always the cause of a symptom. Further, some symptoms are caused by several factors. Causal factors include

- cancer
- treatment
- debility
- concurrent disorder.

Treatment depends on the underlying pathological mechanism

Even when the cancer is responsible, a symptom may be caused in different ways, e.g. vomiting from hypercalcaemia and vomiting from raised intracranial pressure. Treatment will vary accordingly.

Explanation

Explain the underlying mechanism(s) in simple terms

Treatment begins with an explanation by the doctor of the reason(s) for the symptom. This knowledge does much to reduce the psychological impact of the symptom on the sufferer, e.g. 'The shortness of breath is caused partly by the cancer itself and partly by fluid at the base of the right lung. In addition, you are anaemic.'

If explanation is omitted, the patient may continue to think that his condition is shrouded in mystery. This is frightening because 'even the doctors don't know what's going on'.

Discuss treatment options with the patient

Whenever possible, the doctor and the patient should decide together on the immediate course of action. Few things are more damaging to a person's self-esteem than to be excluded from discussions about one's self.

Individualized treatment

Do not limit treatment to the use of drugs

- treatment may be physical or psychological or both
- treatment may be drug or nondrug or both.

For example, pruritus is relieved in the majority of patients without resort to antihistamines. Aqueous cream applied to dry, itching skin several times a day and soap eliminated in favour of emulsifying ointment is frequently sufficient.

Prescribe drugs prophylactically for persistent symptoms

When treating a persistent symptom with a drug, it should be administered regularly on a prophylactic basis. The use of drugs as needed instead of regularly is the cause of much unrelieved distress.

Keep the treatment as simple as possible

When an additional drug is considered, ask the following questions:

'What is the treatment goal?'

'How can it be monitored?'

'What is the risk of adverse effects?'

'What is the risk of drug interactions?'

'Is it possible to stop any of the current medication?'

Seek a colleague's advice in seemingly intractable situations

No one can be an expert in all aspects of patient care. For example, the management of an unusual genito-urinary problem is likely to be enhanced by advice from a urologist or gynaecologist.

Never say 'I have tried everything' or 'There is nothing more I can do'

It is generally possible to develop a repertoire of alternative measures. Although it is wise not to promise too much, it is important to re-assure the patient that you are going to stand by him and do all you can to help, e.g. 'No promises but we'll do our best.'

Instead of attempting immediately to relieve a symptom completely, be prepared to chip away at the problem a little at a time. When tackled in this way it is surprising how much can be achieved with determination and persistence.

Written advice is essential

Precise guidelines are necessary to achieve maximum patient co-operation. 'Take as much as you like, as often as you like' is a recipe for anxiety, poor symptom relief and maximum adverse effects. The drug regimen should be written out in full for the patient and his family to work from. Times to be taken, names of drugs, reason for use (for pain, for bowels etc.) and dose (x ml, y tablets) should all be stated. Also there should be details of what to do when medication runs out.

Supervision

Review! Review! Review!

It is often difficult to predict the optimum dose of a symptom relief drug, particularly opioids, laxatives and psychotropic drugs. Further, adverse effects put drug compliance in jeopardy. Arrangements must be made for continuing supervision and adjustment of medication.

It is sometimes necessary to compromise on complete relief in order to avoid unacceptable adverse effects. For example, anticholinergic effects such as dry mouth or visual disturbance may limit dose escalation. With inoperable bowel obstruction it may be better to aim to reduce the incidence of vomiting to once or twice a day rather than to seek complete relief.

Cancer is a progressive disease and new symptoms occur. These must be dealt with urgently.

Attention to detail

'Thou shalt not make assumptions.'

'To *ass-u-me* is to make an *ass* of *u* and *me*.'[31]

Attention to detail requires an inquisitive mind, one which repeatedly asks why:

'Why is this patient with breast cancer vomiting? She is not taking morphine; she is not hypercalcaemic. Why is she vomiting?'

'This patient with cancer of the pancreas has pain in the neck. It does not fit with the usual pattern of metastatic spread. Why does he have pain there?'

Attention to detail is important at every stage – in evaluation, explanation (e.g. avoid jargon, use simple language) and when planning and prescribing treatment (e.g. preparing written advice and drug regimens which are easy to follow).

Attention to detail makes all the difference to palliative care – without it success may be forfeited and patients suffer needlessly.

Pain

'Pain is what the patient says hurts.'

Pain is an unpleasant *sensory* and *emotional* experience associated with actual or potential tissue damage or described in terms of such damage.[32] In other words, pain is a *somatopsychic* phenomenon. The perception of pain is modulated by

- the patient's *mood*
- the patient's *morale*
- the *meaning* of the pain for the patient.

The meaning of persistent pain in advanced cancer is 'I am incurable, I am going to die'. Other factors affecting pain threshold are shown in Table 3.1. Because of the multidimensional nature of pain, it is often helpful to think in terms of total pain, encompassing the physical, psychological, social and spiritual aspects of suffering.

People with chronic pain generally do not look in pain because of the absence of autonomic concomitants (Table 3.2). In cancer, acute pain concomitants may be evident particularly if the pain is severe and of recent onset or paroxysmal.

Table 3.1   Factors affecting pain threshold

Threshold lowered	Threshold raised
Discomfort	Relief of other symptoms
Insomnia	Sleep
Fatigue	Sympathy
Anxiety	Understanding
Fear	Companionship
Anger	Creative activity
Sadness	Relaxation
Depression	Reduction in anxiety
Boredom	Elevation of mood
Mental isolation	Analgesics
Social abandonment	Anxiolytics
	Antidepressants

Table 3.2   Temporal classification of pain

	Acute	Chronic	
Time course	Transient	Persistent	
Meaning to patient	Positive draws attention to injury or illness	Negative serves no useful purpose	Positive as patient obtains secondary gain
Concomitants	Fight or flight pupillary dilatation increased sweating tachypnoea tachycardia shunting of blood from viscera to muscles	Vegetative sleep disturbance anorexia decreased libido no pleasure in life constipation somatic pre-occupation personality change lethargy	

Because of the implications for treatment, it is also important to distinguish between pain caused by stimulation of nerve endings (nociceptive pain) and pain caused by nerve dysfunction (neuropathic pain). Neuropathic pain is often only partially responsive to treatment with standard analgesics, including morphine and other opioids (see p.72). Thus, from a therapeutic point of view, it is often helpful to think of pain in cancer in terms of the response to opioids (Table 3.3):

Opioid responsive, i.e. pain relieved by opioids

Opioid semiresponsive, i.e. pain relieved by the concurrent use of an opioid and an adjuvant drug (co-analgesic)

Opioid resistant, i.e. pain not relieved by opioids.

Opioid resistance may be more apparent than real (Table 3.4). Painful muscle spasm (cramp) is a good example of true opioid resistant pain. Cramp in various parts of the body is relatively common in cancer. It is often associated with bone pain which is exacerbated by movement. Anxiety is also a potent exacerbating factor (Figure 3.1).

Myofascial pain is a specific form of cramp. Myofascial trigger points occur most commonly in the pectoral girdle and neck.

Table 3.3 Types of pain and implications for treatment

Type of pain	Mechanism	Example	Response to opioids	Treatment
Nociceptive visceral somatic muscle spasm	Stimulation of nerve endings	Hepatic capsule pain Bone pain	+ +/– –	Analgesics Analgesics Muscle relaxant
Neuropathic nerve compression	Stimulation of nervi nervorum (?)		+/–	Analgesics; corticosteroid
nerve injury	Peripheral nerve injury (de-afferentation pain)	Neuroma or nerve infiltration (e.g. brachial or lumbo-sacral plexus)	(+)/–	Trial of opioid; trial of corticosteroid; tricyclic antidepressant; anticonvulsant; local anaesthetic congener; spinal analgesia; ketamine; TENS
	CNS injury	Spinal cord compression or post-stroke pain		
sympathetically maintained	Abnormal sympathetic activity	Causalgia	–	Sympathetic nerve block

Table 3.4   Opioid resistant cancer pain: clinical classification

Pseudoresistant

Underdosing
Poor alimentary absorption (rare)
Poor alimentary absorption because of vomiting
Ignoring psychological aspects of care

Semiresistant/semiresponsive

Soft tissue
Muscle infiltration   } associated with local inflammation
Bone metastasis
Neuropathic (some)
Raised intracranial pressure
Movement related

Resistant

Neuropathic (some)
Muscle spasm

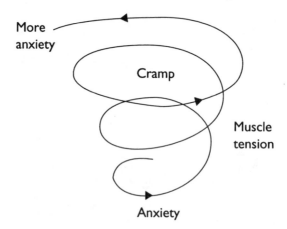

Figure 3.1   Relationship between anxiety and cramp.

Pain in advanced cancer

Pain and advanced cancer are not synonymous

- three quarters of patients experience pain
- one quarter of patients do not experience pain.

Multiple concurrent pains are common in those who have pain

- about one third has a single pain
- one third has two pains
- one third has three or more pains.[33]

Pain in cancer can be grouped into four causal categories

- caused by cancer itself (85% of patients)
- caused by treatment (17%)
- related to cancer and/or debility (9%)
- caused by a concurrent disorder (9%).[33]

Common individual causes are shown below (Table 3.5).

Table 3.5   Top 10 pains in patients with advanced cancer at Sobell House (n = 211)

1 Bone	
2 Visceral	caused by cancer itself
3 Neuropathic	
4 Soft tissue	
5 Immobility	
6 Constipation	
7 Myofascial	related to cancer and/or debility
8 Cramp	
9 Oesophagitis	
10 Degeneration of the spine	concurrent disorder

Pain management

Pain relief is often achieved by adopting a broad-spectrum (i.e. multimodal) approach (Table 3.6).

If anticancer treatment is recommended, analgesics should be given until the treatment ameliorates the pain – which may take several weeks.

Table 3.6   Pain management in cancer

Examination
 	
To establish trust
To confirm site
To identify cause
 	
Explanation to reduce psychological impact of pain
 	
Modification of pathological process
 	
Radiation therapy
Hormone therapy
Chemotherapy
Surgery
 	
Analgesics
 	
Primary
  nonopioids
  opioids
Secondary
  corticosteroids
  antidepressants
  anticonvulsants
  muscle relaxants
 	
Nondrug methods
 	
Physical
  heat pads
  transcutaneous electrical nerve
    stimulation (TENS)
	Psychological
	  relaxation
	  cognitive-behavioural therapy
	  psychodynamic therapy
	
	Interruption of pain pathways
	
	Local anaesthesia
	  lignocaine
	  bupivacaine
	Neurolysis
	  chemical (alcohol, phenol,
	    chlorocresol)
	  cold (cryotherapy)
	  heat (thermocoagulation)
	Neurosurgery
	  cervical spinothalamic
	    tractotomy (cordotomy)
	
	Modification of way of life and environment
	
	Avoid pain-precipitating activities
	Immobilization of the painful part
	  cervical collar
	  surgical corset
	  slings
	  orthopaedic surgery
	Walking aid
	Wheelchair
	Hoist

Since the advent of spinal analgesia (*see* p.76), neurolytic and neurosurgical procedures have become almost obsolete in the UK. At many centres, coeliac axis plexus block with alcohol for epigastric visceral pain is the only neurolytic block still used.

Some patients continue to experience pain on movement despite analgesics, other drugs, radiotherapy and nerve blocks. Here, the situation is often improved by suggesting modifications to the patient's way of life and environment. This is where the help of a physiotherapist and an occupational therapist is often invaluable.

It is generally best to aim at progressive pain relief

- relief at night
- relief at rest during the day
- relief on movement (not always completely possible).

Relief should be evaluated in relation to each pain. If there is severe anxiety and/or depression, it may take 3–4 weeks to achieve maximum benefit. Re-evaluation is a continuing necessity; old pains may get worse and new ones develop.

Principles of analgesic use

For pain caused by the cancer itself, drugs generally give adequate relief provided the right drug is administered in the right dose at the right time intervals.

By the mouth

The oral route is the preferred route for analgesics, including morphine and other strong opioids.

By the clock

Persistent pain requires preventive therapy. Analgesics should be given regularly and prophylactically. As needed medication is irrational and inhumane.

By the ladder

Use a 3-step analgesic ladder (Figure 3.2). If a drug fails to relieve, *move up the ladder*; do not move laterally in the same efficacy group.

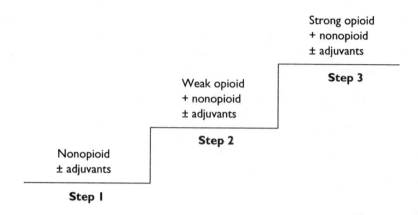

Figure 3.2   The World Health Organization 3-step analgesic ladder.[34]

Table 3.7   Adjuvant drugs for analgesic ladder

Control of adverse effects	*Secondary analgesics*
Laxative	Corticosteroid
Anti-emetic	Antidepressant
	Anticonvulsant
Psychotropic medication	Muscle relaxant
Night sedative	
Anxiolytic	
Antidepressant	

Individual treatment

The right dose of an analgesic is the dose which relieves the pain.

Supervision

The response to treatment must be monitored to ensure that benefits of treatment are maximized and adverse effects minimized.

Adjuvant drugs

A laxative is almost always necessary with an opioid; about 50% of patients need an anti-emetic (Table 3.7).

Nonopioids

The main nonopioids are

- aspirin
- other nonsteroidal anti-inflammatory drugs (NSAIDs)
- paracetamol/acetaminophen.

Nonopioids are step 1 analgesics. Because of their anti-inflammatory effect, NSAIDs are particularly useful for metastatic bone and soft tissue pains. They should be used even when a strong opioid is also necessary.

In hot countries, NSAIDs are sometimes discouraged because of the risk of acute renal failure in hypovolaemic patients. Paracetamol is used instead.

Mode of action

Nonopioids inhibit prostaglandin (PG) synthesis by inhibiting the enzyme cyclo-oxygenase (COX). They do this to a variable extent in different tissues. Paracetamol inhibits PG synthesis in the brain but has no effect on PG synthesis in inflamed joints. Thus, although paracetamol is analgesic and antipyretic (like the NSAIDs), it is not anti-inflammatory in rheumatoid arthritis. The relative benefits of the NSAIDs and paracetamol in painful bone metastases has yet to be determined.

COX exists in two forms. COX-1 is constitutive (i.e. present in all normal tissues), whereas COX-2 is normally undetectable in most tissues but massively induced by inflammation. By producing selective COX-2 inhibitors, it is hoped to reduce the gastric toxicity of NSAIDs.

Inhibition of PG synthesis does not account for the total analgesic effect of NSAIDs, although it appears to explain most of the adverse effects. In post-dental extraction pain, most weak COX inhibitors are significantly superior to aspirin and most strong inhibitors inferior. Ketorolac is an example of a weak COX inhibitor which is superior to aspirin and most other NSAIDs in terms of analgesic efficacy.

Nonopioids and platelet function

- aspirin causes *irreversible* impairment of platelet function (with prolongation of bleeding time) by inactivating platelet COX permanently by acetylation
- most other NSAIDs cause reversible impairment of platelet function

- *nonacetylated salicylates* have no effect on platelet function at normal therapeutic doses:
  choline magnesium salicylate
  diflunisal
  salsalate

- meloxicam, a COX-1 sparing NSAID, also has no effect on platelet function.[35]

Common adverse effects and interactions

- gastric erosions, peptic ulcers, haemorrhage:
  more with cheap standard aspirin tablets because of coarse granular nature
  less with dispersible and enteric-coated aspirin, comparable to other NSAIDs
  ibuprofen (available 'over the counter') is least toxic in this respect

- many NSAIDs *and paracetamol* induce bronchospasm in susceptible patients; *choline salicylate, choline magnesium trisalicylate, azapropazone and benzydamine do not*

- aspirin may cause tinnitus and deafness, particularly in hypo-albuminaemic patients

- all NSAIDs cause salt and water retention which may result in ankle oedema. In consequence, they *antagonize* the action of diuretics to a variable extent

- aspirin *potentiates* oral hypoglycaemic agents

- aspirin *antagonizes* uricosuric agents.

Distinguishing features of paracetamol

- it can be taken by most patients who are hypersensitive to aspirin; cross-sensitivity occurs in only 25%

- it does not injure the gastric mucosa

- it is well tolerated by patients with peptic ulcers

- it does not affect plasma uric acid concentration

- it has no effect on platelet function

- liquid preparations are stable

- adverse effects are uncommon.

The main drawback with paracetamol is the frequency of administration (q4h–q6h). Because NSAIDs are mainly peripheral in action and paracetamol central, the two can be used in combination with an additive effect.

Choice of NSAID

This depends on several factors, e.g. availability, fashion, cost, frequency of administration, individual toxicity and response. Typical regimens include:

Ibuprofen	400–600 mg q.d.s.
Flurbiprofen	50–100 mg b.d.
Naproxen	250–500 mg b.d.
Diflunisal	250–500 mg b.d.
Diclofenac (m/r)	150–200 mg o.d.
Benorylate suspension	5–10 ml b.d.

Weak opioids

Weak opioids in combination with nonopioids are step 2 analgesics (Table 3.8). A weak opioid is as effective as a small dose of morphine. This means that step 2 is pharmacologically unnecessary. In many countries, however, it is much easier to obtain and supply a weak opioid preparation.

Codeine is a prodrug of morphine. It is about 1/10 as potent as morphine. *About 10% of the population cannot convert codeine to morphine.* The typical dose range for codeine is 30–60 mg q4h. Dihydrocodeine is generally used instead in the UK.

Table 3.8   Commonly used weak opioid compound preparations (UK)

	Drug content	
Generic name	Weak opioid	Nonopioid
Co-codaprin 8/400	Codeine 8 mg	Aspirin 400 mg
Co-codamol 8/500	Codeine 8 mg	Paracetamol 500 mg
Co-codamol 30/500	Codeine 30 mg	Paracetamol 500 mg
Co-dydramol 10/500	Dihydrocodeine 10 mg	Paracetamol 500 mg
Co-proxamol 32.5/325	Dextropropoxyphene hydrochloride 32.5 mg	Paracetamol 325 mg

Tramadol

Tramadol is an alternative opioid for both step 2 and the lower end of step 3. Its exact relative potency with oral codeine and oral morphine in cancer patients is still debatable. By injection, it is 1/10 as potent as morphine. In Table 3.9 (*see* p.69) it is regarded as double strength codeine, i.e. 1/5 strength morphine. This difference relates to the high oral bio-availability of tramadol (about 70%).

Tramadol has a dual mechanism of analgesic action, part opioid and part a presynaptic re-uptake blocker of mono-amines (like a tricyclic antidepressant; *see* p.78). It does not have anticholinergic or antidepressant properties. The dual analgesic action is synergistic. Adverse opioid effects are significantly less than with codeine and morphine.

There is circumstantial evidence that tramadol lowers seizure threshold. Patients with a history of epilepsy should generally *not* be prescribed tramadol. Tramadol should be used with caution, if at all, in patients taking other medication which lowers seizure threshold, notably tricyclic antidepressants and SSRIs.

Strong opioids

These are step 3 analgesics. As in step 2, a nonopioid should normally be given concurrently.

Morphine and other strong opioids exist to be given, not merely to be withheld. Their use is dictated by therapeutic need, not by brevity of prognosis.

Morphine does not cause clinically important respiratory depression in cancer patients in pain. This is because *pain is a physiological antagonist to the central depressant effects of morphine.* Thus, it is extremely rare to need to use naloxone, a specific opioid antagonist, in palliative care. Further, in contrast to postoperative patients, cancer patients with pain

- have generally been receiving a weak opioid for some time, i.e. are not opioid naive
- take medication by mouth (slower absorption, lower peak concentration)
- titrate the dose upwards step by step (less likelihood of an excessive dose being given).

The relationship of the therapeutic dose to the lethal dose of morphine (the therapeutic ratio) is greater than commonly supposed. Patients who take a double dose of morphine at bedtime (*see* below) are no more likely to die during the night than those who do not.

Morphine is metabolized mainly to morphine-3-glucuronide and morphine-6-glucuronide. The former is inactive, whereas the latter is *more* potent as an analgesic than morphine itself. Both glucuronides cumulate in renal failure. This results in a prolonged duration of action for morphine, with a danger of severe sedation and subsequent respiratory depression if the dose and/or frequency of administration are not reduced.

Tolerance to morphine is not a practical problem. Psychological dependence (addiction) does not occur if morphine is used correctly. Physical dependence does not prevent a reduction in the dose of morphine if the patient's pain ameliorates, e.g. as a result of radiotherapy or a nerve block.

Morphine is not the panacea for cancer pain. Its use does not guarantee success, particularly if the psychosocial aspects of care are ignored.

Oral morphine

Morphine by mouth is the strong opioid of choice for cancer pain. It is administered as tablets (10 mg, 20 mg), in aqueous solutions (e.g. 2 mg in 1 ml), as m/r tablets (5 mg, 10 mg, 15 mg, 30 mg, 60 mg, 100 mg, 200 mg), or in a m/r suspension.

If the patient was previously receiving a weak opioid, begin with 10 mg q4h (or m/r 30 mg q12h). With frail elderly patients, consider starting on 5 mg q4h in order to reduce initial drowsiness, confusion and unsteadiness.

If changing from an alternative strong opioid (e.g. buprenorphine, levorphanol, methadone), a much higher dose of morphine may be needed (Table 3.9, p.69).

The patient should be encouraged to take additional rescue doses if the pain is not adequately relieved or returns before the next regular dose is due.

Adjust the dose upwards after 24 h if the pain is not 90% relieved (e.g. 5 → 10 mg, 10 → 15 mg, 20 → 30 mg). Two thirds of patients never need more than 30 mg q4h (or m/r morphine 100 mg q12h). The rest need up to 200 mg q4h (or m/r morphine 600 mg q12h) and occasionally more.

With ordinary tablets or solution, a double dose at bedtime usually enables a patient to go through the night without waking in pain.

Morphine should generally be given together with a nonopioid.

Supply an anti-emetic for regular use should nausea or vomiting develop, e.g. haloperidol 1.5 mg stat and nocte.

Prescribe laxatives, e.g. co-danthrusate or senna + docusate. Adjust dose according to response. Suppositories and enemas continue to be necessary in about one third of patients. *Constipation may be more difficult to manage than the pain.*

Warn patients about the possibility of initial drowsiness.

Write out the drug regimen in detail with times, names of drugs and amount to be taken; arrange for follow-up.

If swallowing is difficult or vomiting persists, morphine may be given PR by suppository (same dose as PO). Alternatively, give half of the oral dose of morphine by SC injection or one third of the oral dose as SC diamorphine.

Diamorphine

Diamorphine hydrochloride (di-acetylmorphine, heroin) is available for medicinal use only in the UK and Canada. It is much more soluble than morphine sulphate/hydrochloride and is used in the UK instead of morphine when injections are necessary because large amounts can be given in very small volumes.

By injection, diamorphine is twice as potent as morphine. By this route, its initial effects are mediated by the primary metabolite, mono-acetylmorphine.

Because of rapid de-acetylation, diamorphine by mouth is merely a prodrug for morphine. Possibly because of better absorption (it is highly lipid soluble), it is slightly more potent than morphine by this route.

Converting from morphine to diamorphine or changing routes

The following conversion ratios are approximate and should be regarded only as a general guide[36]

- oral morphine to SC morphine, halve the oral dose
- oral morphine to IV morphine, give one third of the oral dose
- oral morphine to SC diamorphine, give one third of the oral dose
- oral diamorphine to SC diamorphine, halve the oral dose.

When changing from either oral diamorphine or oral morphine to m/r morphine, convert 1 mg for 1 mg and adjust as necessary.

There are no generic m/r morphine tablets. Because of differing pharmacokinetic profiles, it may be best to keep individual patients on the same brand.

Improving drug compliance

Because most wards have only four drug rounds a day (0600, 1200, 1800 and 2200 h), special provision has to be made to enable a patient to receive morphine q4h. In practice, the interval between the first drug round (0600 h) and the last (2200 h) is usually less than 16 h, and it is not uncommon to see a series of entries such as:

0725, 1125, 1550, 2130 h
0725, 1125, 1525, 1925, 2350 h

In the first example, it proved impossible to give the third dose on time and the fourth has been delayed partly for convenience and partly to 'help you have a better night'. In the second example, the nurses have coped with a highly individual regimen until bedtime, but then 'Here is your night sedative, Mr Smith. You cannot have your morphine yet, it's not due. We'll bring it later'.

The patient either fails to get to sleep because of worry about the pain returning or complains bitterly when woken from a deep sleep by a nurse an hour or so later. In both instances, the comfort (and sleep) of the patient is put in jeopardy by a pharisaical attitude to the concept of 'every four hours'.

It is often necessary to catch up at some stage in the day. Catching up is best done at 1000 h. If 'time slippage' occurs later in the day, catching up should be repeated, preferably at the next administration and certainly at 2200 h.

The interval between the early morning dose and the 1000 h dose is generally less than four hours, occasionally less than three. The nurses should be advised specifically on this point.

When catching up is practised, it is much easier for the nurses to administer medication q4h. In fact, the only administration in addition to the routine q.d.s. drug rounds is 1000 h. This is a time when the maximum number of nurses are available, and when Controlled Drug book-keeping is easiest to complete.

Check daily to ensure that all the prescribed doses have been given.

Most patients given a double dose at bedtime of ordinary morphine tablets or solution will sleep painfree through the night.

Additional rescue doses of morphine should be prescribed for breakthrough pain. Instructions must be clear: extra morphine does not mean that the next dose of regular morphine is omitted.

If extra morphine is requested several times a day, it is an indication that the regular dose needs to be adjusted upwards.

The availability of m/r tablets has simplified considerably the use of morphine on general wards.

Alternative strong opioids

There are multiple opioid receptor subtypes in many areas of the CNS, including the dorsal horn of the spinal cord. Mu, kappa and delta opioid receptors are all involved in analgesia. Opioids differ from each other in terms of intrinsic activity and receptor site affinity. This property can be utilized in patients who are intolerant of morphine (mainly a mu agonist) by converting, for example, to methadone (a mixed mu and delta agonist).

When converting from an alternative strong opioid to oral morphine, the initial dose depends on the relative potency of the two drugs (Table 3.9). Table 3.9 should also be used to determine an appropriate starting dose of an alternative opioid in someone intolerant of morphine (marked dysphoria and/or sedation, hallucinations, nausea and vomiting, pruritus, which fail to respond to appropriate measures).

Pethidine and dextromoramide have little place in cancer pain management because of short durations of action. Some centres use dextromoramide for breakthrough pain in patients taking regular morphine, or as prophylactic additional analgesia before a painful dressing or other procedure. This is because of its rapid onset of action. Generally, patients obtain satisfactory relief from an additional dose of morphine or by timing the procedure for one hour after a regular dose.

Pentazocine should not be used; it is a weak opioid by mouth and often causes psychotomimetic effects (dysphoria, depersonalization, frightening dreams, hallucinations).

Methadone

Methadone is a mixed mu and delta opioid agonist and a NMDA receptor antagonist.[37] Some patients with nociceptive pain who obtain only poor relief with morphine but severe adverse effects (drowsiness, delirium, nausea and vomiting) obtain good relief with methadone at a lower equivalent dose with few or no adverse effects.

At Sobell House, methadone is used mainly in selected patients with renal failure who have developed excessive drowsiness and/or delirium with morphine because of cumulation of morphine-6-glucuronide. Methadone does not have a comparable active metabolite and its effects are therefore not altered in renal failure.

Table 3.9   Approximate oral analgesic equivalence to morphine[a]

Analgesic	Potency ratio with morphine	Duration of action (h)[b]
Codeine ⎫ Dihydrocodeine ⎭	1/10	3–5
Pethidine (meperidine USA)	1/8	2–3
Tramadol	1/5[c]	5–6
Dipipanone (in Diconal UK)	1/2	3–5
Papaveretum	2/3[d]	3–5
Oxycodone	4/3[c]	5–6
Dextromoramide	2[e]	2–3
Levorphanol	5	6–8
Phenazocine	5	6–8
Methadone	5–10[f]	8–12
Hydromorphone	8	3–5
Buprenorphine (*sublingual*)	60	6–8
Fentanyl (*transdermal*)	150	72

a   multiply dose of opioid by its potency ratio to determine the equivalent dose of morphine sulphate

b   dependent in part on severity of pain and on dose; often longer lasting in very elderly and those with renal dysfunction

c   tramadol and oxycodone are both relatively more potent by mouth because of high bio-availability; parenteral potency ratios with morphine are 1/10 and 3/4 respectively

d   papaveretum (strong opium) is standardized to contain 50% morphine base; potency expressed in relation to morphine sulphate

e   dextromoramide: a single 5 mg dose is equivalent to morphine 15 mg in terms of peak effect but is shorter acting; overall potency ratio adjusted accordingly

f   methadone: by injection, a single 5 mg dose is equivalent to morphine 7.5 mg. However, its long plasma halflife and its broad-spectrum receptor affinity results in a much higher than expected potency ratio when given repeatedly.[38]

The plasma halflife of methadone ranges from 8–80 h and is affected by changes in urinary pH. Cumulation is a potential problem for most patients. Dose titration is therefore different from morphine. For 2–3 days patients are advised to take a dose *q3h as needed*; after this most patients can be converted to either a b.d. or t.d.s. regimen.

Hydromorphone

Hydromorphone is an analogue of morphine with similar pharmacokinetic and pharmacodynamic properties. By mouth it is some 8 times more potent than morphine; by injection 5–6 times. As with morphine, there is wide interpatient variation in bio-availability.

Fentanyl

Fentanyl, like morphine, is mainly a strong mu agonist. It is widely used as a peri-operative analgesic. Transdermal patches (TTS-fentanyl) are available for cancer pain management. These deliver 25, 50, 75 or 100 mcg/h over 3 days. Patients who have not previously taken morphine or other strong opioids should always be started on the lowest dose, i.e. 25 mcg/h.

Peak plasma concentrations of fentanyl are achieved after 12–24 h and a depot remains in the skin for some 24 h after the patch is removed. A few patients obtain relief for only 48 h rather than the intended 72 h. High fever and exposure of transdermal patches to external heat sources (e.g. heat pads, electric blankets) may increase the rate of delivery of fentanyl.

The patches do not permit rapid dose titration because of the slow onset of activity. Rescue medication with morphine will be necessary during the first 24 h. The effective dose varies widely because of differences in pain intensity and variability in the metabolism and excretion of fentanyl. A reduction of laxative medication is generally necessary.

Buprenorphine

Buprenorphine is a potent partial mu agonist, kappa antagonist and delta agonist. It is an alternative to oral morphine in the low to middle part of morphine's dose range. In low doses, buprenorphine and morphine are additive in their effects; at very high doses, antagonism by buprenorphine may occur. There is no need, however, to prescribe both. Use one or the other.

Buprenorphine is available as a *sublingual* tablet; ingestion reduces bio-availability. It needs to be given only q8h. With daily doses of over 3 mg, patients may prefer to take fewer tablets q6h.

It is generally considered that there is an analgesic ceiling at a daily dose of 3–5 mg; equivalent to 180–300 mg of oral morphine/24 h. In some countries, 1.6 mg is regarded as the ceiling daily dose. Whether this represents genetic differences or local custom is not clear.

Buprenorphine is not an alternative to codeine or other weak opioid. Like morphine, it should be used when a weak opioid has failed. Assuming the previous regular use of a weak opioid, patients should commence on 200 mcg q8h with the advice that, 'If it is not more effective than your previous tablets take a further 200 mcg after 1 h, and 400 mcg q8h after that.'

When changing to morphine, multiply the total daily dose of buprenorphine by 60. If the pain was previously poorly relieved, multiply by 100. Adverse effects, e.g. nausea, vomiting, constipation, drowsiness, need to be monitored as with morphine.

Continuous subcutaneous infusions

When oral administration is no longer feasible, continuous SC infusion of morphine sulphate, diamorphine hydrochloride or hydromorphone obviates the need for injections q4h (Table 3.10).

Table 3.10   Drugs given by SC infusion

Commonly used	Occasionally used	Not suitable
Diamorphine	Diclofenac[b]	Prochlorperazine[e]
Morphine	Ketorolac[b]	Diazepam[e]
Hydromorphone	Dexamethasone[c]	
Metoclopramide	Levomepromazine	
Cyclizine[a]	Chlorpromazine[a]	
Haloperidol	Phenobarbital[d]	
Hyoscine butylbromide		
Hyoscine hydrobromide		
Midazolam		

a   tends to cause local SC inflammation
b   immiscible with other drugs except diamorphine in saline
c   no advantage over SC injection o.d.
d   immiscible with other drugs except diamorphine and hyoscine
e   too irritant for SC use.

Indications for use

● intractable vomiting

- severe dysphagia
- patient too weak to swallow oral drugs
- poor alimentary absorption (rare).

Advantages

- constant analgesia (no peaks or troughs)
- usually reloaded once in 24 h
- comfort and confidence (no repeated injections)
- does not limit mobility
- permits better control of nausea and vomiting.

Choice of infusion sites

- upper chest (intercostal plane)
- upper arm (outer aspect)
- abdomen
- thighs.

If the infusion causes painful local inflammation, consider

- changing the needle site prophylactically, e.g. daily
- reducing the quantity of the irritant drug
- changing to an alternative drug, e.g. cyclizine to hyoscine
- giving the irritant drug IM or PR
- adding hydrocortisone sodium succinate 25–50 mg to the syringe.

Neuropathic pain

Definition

Neuropathic pain is pain associated with neuropathy, i.e. nerve compression and nerve injury (somatic, visceral, sympathetic) or CNS lesions. Pain in an area of abnormal or absent sensation is always neuropathic.

Pathogenesis

There are many causes of neuropathic pain in cancer (Table 3.11). Such pain stems from three different mechanisms.

Table 3.11   Causes of neuropathic pain in advanced cancer

Caused by cancer	Related to cancer and/or debility
Nerve compression/infiltration Plexopathy Spinal cord compression Thalamic tumour	Postherpetic neuralgia *Concurrent causes*
Caused by treatment	Diabetic neuropathy Poststroke pain
Postoperative incisional pain Phantom limb pain Chemotherapy (peripheral neuropathy) Radiation (brachial plexopathy)	

Nerve compression

For example, nerve root compression caused by a collapsed vertebra.

Nerve injury

For example, brachial and lumbosacral plexus infiltration by cancer. This may evolve from earlier nerve compression.

Nerve injury causes pain as a result of

- neuronal hyperexcitability:
  spontaneous activity
  mechanical sensitivity
  α adrenergic sensitivity
- a cascade of neurochemical and physiological changes in the CNS, particularly in the dorsal horn of the spinal cord.

Nerve injury does not always lead to pain, e.g. postherpetic neuralgia is rare in young people. Further, with identical lesions, only a minority develops pain. A genetic factor has been postulated.

Sympathetically maintained pain

This is an uncommon form of neuropathic pain, related to sympathetic nerve trauma at operation or 'irritation' by a tumour. It is similar to somatic nerve injury pain but has an arterial distribution instead of a neurodermatomal one. It differs also in its response to treatment.

Clinical features of nerve injury pain

Distribution

Neurodermatomal, if peripheral lesion.

Quality

Superficial burning/stinging pain, particularly if peripheral lesion; +/– spontaneous stabbing/shooting pain. There may also be a deep aching component.

Concomitants

- often receiving morphine with little effect; often exhausted because of insomnia
- allodynia (light touch exacerbates pain); unable to bear clothing against affected area
- sensory deficit, e.g. numbness
- sometimes there is a sympathetic component manifesting as autonomic instability, i.e. cutaneous vasodilation, increased skin temperature, changes in sweating pattern.

Management

Explanation

Nerve compression pain

'Needs cortisone as well as painkillers.'

Nerve injury pain

'Often does not respond well to painkillers such as aspirin and morphine.'

'Need to start a different type of painkiller.'

'First step is to get a good night's sleep.'

Drugs of choice

Nerve compression pain

A combination of morphine and a corticosteroid, e.g. dexamethasone 4–8 mg o.d., is often effective (Figure 3.3).

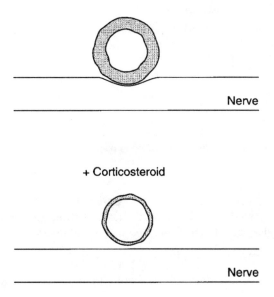

Figure 3.3   Possible mechanism of action of corticosteroids in relief of nerve compression pain. Total tumour mass = neoplasm + surrounding inflammation. General anti-inflammatory effect of corticosteroid reduces total tumour mass resulting in reduction of pain.

Nerve injury pain

This is often relatively resistant to morphine and corticosteroids. When this is so, it is necessary to use one or more secondary analgesics, i.e. drugs not marketed primarily as analgesics but of proven value in relieving nerve injury pain (Figure 3.4).

- as a general rule, use a tricyclic antidepressant for superficial burning pain and allodynia

- as a general rule, use an anticonvulsant for spontaneous stabbing/shooting pain

- if both types of pain are present, use *either* an antidepressant *or* an anticonvulsant (step 1) before proceeding to both (step 2)

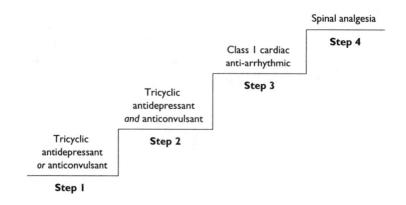

Figure 3.4   An analgesic ladder for nerve injury pain.

- some centres use a class 1 cardiac anti-arrhythmic, e.g. flecainide or mexiletine – styled step 3 here – as the drug of choice for nerve injury pain, i.e. it is used as step 1. These are chemically related to local anaesthetics

- other centres move straight from step 2 to step 4 (spinal analgesia)

- spinal analgesia includes both epidural and intrathecal routes

- nerve injury pain is more responsive to spinal morphine than morphine by conventional routes. (Spinal analgesia is also used occasionally in patients with nociceptive pain who experience intolerable adverse effects with PO or SC morphine)

- epidural morphine + bupivacaine +/– clonidine by continuous infusion is one commonly used form of spinal analgesia in cancer patients

- in patients who decline spinal analgesia, ketamine (a dissociative anaesthetic and NMDA receptor antagonist) can be given in subanaesthetic doses by SC infusion

- some patients benefit from transcutaneous electrical nerve stimulation (TENS)

- the putative mechanisms of various secondary analgesics are shown in Figure 3.5.

Sympathetically maintained pain

This responds to sympathetic nerve blocks (stellate ganglion or lumbar sympathetic chain); it does not respond to secondary analgesics.

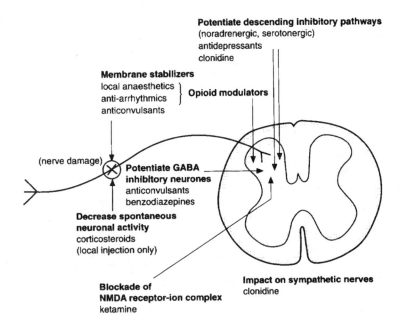

Figure 3.5 Impact of secondary analgesics on peripheral nerves and the dorsal horn of the spinal cord.

Therapeutic guidelines

Tricyclic antidepressant

e.g. amitriptyline 25–75 mg nocte

The rate of increase in dose depends on pain intensity and extent of supervision. Relief may not occur for 4–5 days and is uncommon with only 25 mg. In cancer related neuropathic pain 50–75 mg are generally sufficient. The maximum dose is determined by the degree of relief and by adverse effects. Adverse effects are a common limiting factor. The mechanism of analgesic action is principally by potentiation of descending inhibitory pathways (Figure 3.6).

Anticonvulsant

e.g. sodium valproate 200–1000 mg nocte or carbamazepine

The dose of carbamazepine should be built up slowly from 100 mg b.d. to minimize adverse effects (drowsiness, ataxia, diplopia). Increments should be restricted to 200 mg/week.

● dextropropoxyphene (in co-proxamol) enhances the action of carbamazepine

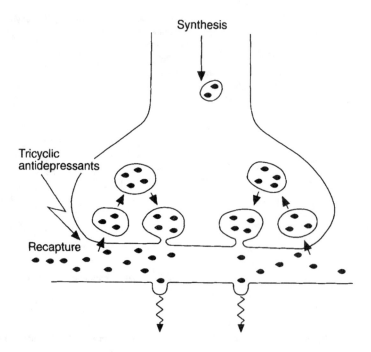

Figure 3.6   Mono-amine neurotransmission at a neuronal synapse (norepinephrine or serotonin/5-hydroxytryptamine). Tricyclics potentiate two descending inhibitory pathways from the brain (one noradrenergic, the other serotonergic) by blocking presynaptic re-uptake. They also potentiate opioid analgesia by a serotonergic mechanism in the brain stem.

- some selective SSRIs increase plasma carbamazepine and plasma valproic acid concentrations; paroxetine does not

- the metabolism of tricyclic antidepressants is accelerated by carbamazepine but, even so, tricyclics antagonize the anticonvulsant action of carbamazepine by lowering the convulsive threshold

- the metabolism of tricyclic antidepressants is inhibited by sodium valproate.

Anti-arrhythmic

e.g. flecainide 50–150 mg b.d. or mexiletine 50–300 mg t.d.s.

The main disadvantage is the negative inotropic effect on the heart. *Should not be given to patients with evidence of cardiac failure.* Toxicity includes confusion, paraesthesiae, multifocal myoclonus, fitting and coma. Use smaller doses in renal failure. Risk of pro-arrhythmic effect if used with a tricyclic.

Expectations

About 75% of patients respond well to step 1–3 drugs; the rest require spinal analgesia or other measures to obtain adequate relief.

The response is not an 'all or none' phenomenon. The crucial first step in many cases is to help the patient obtain a good night's sleep with step 1 or step 2 drugs. The second is to reduce pain intensity and allodynia to a bearable level during the day. Initially, benefit may be for only part of each day. Adverse effects tend to be the limiting therapeutic factor.

The patient should be warned that results often take a week or more to become apparent, although improvement in sleep should occur immediately.

Useful definitions

Pharmacological terms

Receptor affinity ('potency')	A term used to describe the power of attraction between the drug and the drug receptor. Affinity determines the dose of drug required to produce a certain level of biological effect.
Intrinsic activity ('efficacy')	The degree to which the drug is able to stimulate a receptor and thereby produce a biological effect. Intrinsic activity is a basic property of all drugs which act through receptors.
Full agonist	A drug which when bound to the receptor stimulates the receptor to the maximum level, e.g. morphine. By definition the intrinsic activity of a full agonist is unity.
Pure antagonist	A drug which when bound to the receptor fails completely to produce any stimulation of that receptor, e.g. naloxone. By definition the intrinsic activity of a pure antagonist is zero.
Partial agonist	A drug which when bound to the receptor stimulates the receptor to a level below the maximum level, e.g. buprenorphine (partial mu agonist). By definition the intrinsic activity of a partial agonist lies between zero and unity.
Mixed agonist -antagonist	A drug which acts simultaneously on different types of receptor, with the potential for agonist action on one or more types and antagonist action on one or more types, e.g. pentazocine (partial mu agonist + kappa agonist + weak delta antagonist).
Ligand	A substance which binds to a receptor. The use of this term circumvents the need to say whether the substance is an agonist or an antagonist.

Pain terms[32]

Allodynia	Pain caused by a stimulus which does not normally provoke pain.
Anaesthesia dolorosa	Pain in an area which is numb.
Analgesia	Absence of pain in response to stimulation which would normally be painful.
Causalgia	A syndrome of sustained burning pain, allodynia and hyperpathia after a traumatic nerve lesion, often combined with vasomotor and sudomotor dysfunction and later trophic changes.
Central pain	Pain associated with a lesion of the CNS.
Dysaesthesia	An unpleasant abnormal sensation, whether spontaneous or evoked.
Hyperaesthesia	Increased sensitivity to stimulation.
Hyperalgesia	An increased response to a stimulus which is normally painful.
Hyperpathia	A painful syndrome characterized by increased reaction to a stimulus, especially a repetitive stimulus, *as well as an increased threshold*. (This latter feature results in a delayed onset. It tends to be poorly localized and outlasts the stimulus.)
Neuralgia	Pain in the distribution of a nerve.
Neuropathy	A disturbance of function or a pathological change in a nerve.
Nociceptor	A receptor preferentially sensitive to a noxious stimulus or to a stimulus which would become noxious if prolonged.
Noxious stimulus	A noxious stimulus is one which is damaging to normal tissues.
Pain	An unpleasant sensory and emotional experience associated with actual or potential tissue damage or described in terms of such damage.
Pain threshold	The least experience of pain which a subject can recognize.
Pain tolerance level	The greatest level of pain which a subject is prepared to tolerate.

PART FOUR

Symptom Management II

Alimentary symptoms
Respiratory symptoms
Urinary symptoms · Other symptoms
Secondary mental disorders · Drug profiles

Alimentary symptoms

Dyspepsia

Definition

Dyspepsia is postprandial discomfort or pain centred in the upper abdomen (synonym: indigestion).

Pathogenesis

There are many causes of dyspepsia (Table 4.1). From a therapeutic perspective dyspepsia in advanced cancer can be divided into four categories

● small stomach capacity

● gassy

● acid

● dysmotility.

Functional dyspepsia (i.e. dyspepsia without apparent organic cause) is generally caused by dysmotility. It is seen in about 25% of the normal population and is therefore common in patients with cancer.

Most cases of 'squashed stomach syndrome'[39] and 'cancer associated dyspepsia syndrome'[40] are probably examples of functional dysmotility dyspepsia exacerbated by

● opioid induced delayed gastric emptying

● gross hepatomegaly

● gross ascites.

Table 4.1   Causes of dyspepsia in advanced cancer

Caused by cancer	Related to cancer and/or debility
Small stomach capacity	Oesophageal candidiasis
large unresected stomach cancer	Minimal food and fluid intake
linitis plastica	Anxiety → aerophagia
massive ascites	
Gastroparesis (paraneoplastic	Concurrent causes
visceral neuropathy)	
	Organic dyspepsia
Caused by treatment	peptic ulcer
	reflux oesophagitis
Postsurgical	cholelithiasis
postgastrectomy	renal failure
reflux oesophagitis	Non-ulcer dyspepsia
Radiotherapy	dysmotility-like
lumbar spine	aerophagia
epigastrium	
Drugs	
physical irritant (→ gastritis), e.g.	
iron	
metronidazole	
tranexamic acid	
acid stimulant (→ gastritis), e.g.	
NSAIDs	
corticosteroids	
delayed gastric emptying	
anticholinergics	
opioids	
cisplatin	

Evaluation

It is important to differentiate between the four types of dyspepsia because the treatment differs. Careful history taking generally indicates which type is predominant. Patients with dysmotility dyspepsia often have symptoms or a history of irritable bowel syndrome.

Management

Small stomach capacity

If dyspepsia is associated with a small stomach capacity, patients should be advised to separate their main fluid from their main solid intake, and to eat 'small and often', i.e. take five or six small meals/snacks during the day rather than two or three big meals.

Patients with a small stomach capacity may benefit from an antiflatulent after meals – to help clear space in a relatively overfull stomach.

Gassy dyspepsia

Prescribe an antiflatulent, e.g. activated dimeticone. This is available on its own but may conveniently be given in the form of Asilone, a proprietary antacid. Depending on a patient's individual needs, this can be given as needed, q.d.s. or both.

Acid dyspepsia

Prescribe an antacid, an H_2 receptor antagonist (e.g. cimetidine, ranitidine) or a proton pump inhibitor (e.g. omeprazole, lansoprazole).

In patients taking a NSAID, misoprostol (a PG analogue) should be used for dyspepsia, 200 mcg q.d.s. or 400 mcg b.d. If used prophylactically to prevent NSAID gastropathy in patients with a history of peptic ulceration, 200 mcg b.d. is generally adequate.

Dysmotility dyspepsia

This is not helped by gastric acid reduction. Treatment is with a prokinetic drug, i.e. metoclopramide, domperidone, cisapride. These normalize disordered gastric motility.

Nausea and vomiting

There are many potential causes of nausea and vomiting in advanced cancer

● cancer (e.g. bowel obstruction, raised intracranial pressure)

● related to cancer (e.g. hypercalcaemia, constipation)

● treatment (e.g. opioids, NSAIDs, radiotherapy)

● concurrent (e.g. alcoholic gastritis, renal failure).

It is important to identify the most likely cause(s) in each patient because the treatment is dependent on the cause.

On the basis of putative sites of action (Table 4.2), it is possible to derive anti-emetic drugs of choice for different situations (Table 4.3). Anti-emetics must, however, be used appropriately and logically if they are to achieve a satisfactory result (Box 4.A).

Table 4.2   Anti-emetic classification

Putative site or mode of action	Class	Example
Central nervous system		
Vomiting centre	Anticholinergic	Hyoscine hydrobromide, antihistaminic anti-emetics, phenothiazines[a]
	Antihistaminic	Cyclizine, dimenhydrinate, phenothiazines[a]
	$5HT_2$ antagonist	Levomepromazine[b]
Chemoreceptor trigger zone	Dopamine (D_2) antagonist	Haloperidol, droperidol, phenothiazines, metoclopramide, domperidone
Cerebral cortex	Benzodiazepine	Lorazepam
	Cannabinoid	Nabilone
	Corticosteroid	Dexamethasone[c]
Gastro-intestinal tract		
Prokinetic	$5HT_4$ agonist	Metoclopramide, cisapride
	Dopamine (D_2) antagonist	Metoclopramide, domperidone
Vagal $5HT_3$ receptor blockade	$5HT_3$ antagonist	Granisetron, ondansetron, tropisetron
Anti-inflammatory effect	Corticosteroid	Dexamethasone[c]

a   the antihistaminic and anticholinergic properties of phenothiazines vary
b   Levomepromazine is a phenothiazine with $5HT_2$ antagonist properties; this makes it a potent broad-spectrum anti-emetic; its main disadvantages are sedation and postural hypotension
c   the site(s) of action of dexamethasone as an anti-emetic have not been elucidated.

Table 4.3   Choosing an anti-emetic in advanced cancer

Cause of nausea and vomiting	Anti-emetic of choice [alternative]
Drug induced	Haloperidol 1.5–3 mg nocte [Prochlorperazine 5 mg q8h]
Gastric irritation	Treat gastritis; modify medication +/– metoclopramide 10–20 mg q.d.s.
Radiotherapy	Haloperidol 1.5 mg o.d.–b.d.
Chemotherapy	Metoclopramide or 5HT$_3$ receptor antagonist[a] +/– dexamethasone (for doses see BNF, section 4.6)
Metabolic, e.g. hypercalcaemia, uraemia	Haloperidol 5–10 mg nocte or b.d. [5HT$_3$ receptor antagonist][a]
Delayed gastric emptying Functional bowel obstruction	Metoclopramide 10–20 mg q.d.s. [Domperidone 10–20 mg q.d.s.] [Cisapride 20 mg b.d. PO]
Mechanical bowel obstruction	Cyclizine or dimenhydrate 50–100 mg t.d.s. or Hyoscine butylbromide[b] 60–120 mg SC/24 h [Octreotide[b] 300–600 mcg SC/24 h] [5HT$_3$ receptor antagonist][a]
Raised intracranial pressure	Cyclizine or dimenhydrate 50–100 mg t.d.s.
Multifactorial/intractable[c]	Add dexamethasone 8–10 mg o.d. PO/SC or change to levomepromazine 5–12.5 mg SC nocte or 12.5–25 mg PO nocte

a   5HT$_3$ receptor antagonists are beneficial in circumstances in which enterochromaffin cells release excessive amounts of 5HT/serotonin (e.g. chemotherapy, abdominal radiation, abdominal surgery, intestinal distension, renal failure)
b   reduces alimentary secretions and therefore distension and propensity to vomit
c   both dexamethasone and levomepromazine are used as anti-emetics in palliative care 'when all else fails'; a clear order of preference has not been determined.

Box 4.A   Management of nausea and vomiting in palliative care (based on guidelines used at Sir Michael Sobell House, Oxford)

Record severity of the nausea and vomiting, preferably using a formal rating scale.

Document the most likely cause in the patient's case notes.

Treat potentially reversible causes/exacerbating factors, e.g.
constipation
severe pain
coughing
hypercalcaemia (*correction is not always appropriate in dying patients*).

Prescribe first line anti-emetic for the most likely cause (*see* Table 4.3), both *regularly* and *as needed*.

If the patient is vomiting > 3 times in 24 h or within 2 h of taking oral medication, or is nauseated most of the time, administer the anti-emetic parenterally, preferably by continuous SC infusion.

Optimize the dose of anti-emetic every 24 h, taking as needed use into account.

If little or no benefit after 24–48 h despite optimizing the dose, consider:
have you got the cause right?

If no, change to the appropriate anti-emetic and optimize.
If yes, provided the first line anti-emetic has been optimized, add or substitute the second line anti-emetic.

One third of patients with nausea and vomiting need more than one anti-emetic for satisfactory control.

After 72 h of reasonable control using parenteral medication, consider converting to an equivalent oral regimen.

Continue the anti-emetic regimen indefinitely unless the cause is self-limiting.

Anxiety exacerbates nausea and vomiting from any cause and may need specific treatment, either pharmacological or psychological or both.

Constipation

Constipation (difficult defaecation) is common in advanced cancer. Diminished food and fibre intake, lack of exercise and drugs which constipate all contribute to its development. As with nausea and vomiting, it is necessary to be aware of the different classes of laxatives (Table 4.4) and to know which is the laxative of choice in different circumstances.

Patients not on constipating drugs may be satisfactorily treated with senna or bisacodyl tablets. Those receiving morphine often do well with co-danthrusate or co-danthramer, i.e. a combination of a stimulant laxative (danthron) and a softener (Box 4.B).

Table 4.4   Classification of laxatives

Bulk forming drugs (fibre)	*Osmotic laxatives*
Ispaghula husk (Fybogel, Regulan) Methylcellulose Sterculia (Normacol)	Lactulose syrup Magnesium hydroxide suspension (Milk of magnesia) Magnesium sulphate (Epsom salts) Liquid paraffin and magnesium hydroxide oral emulsion BP
Faecal softeners	
Surface wetting agents docusate sodium poloxamer Lubricants liquid paraffin/mineral oil	*Simulant laxatives (colonic)* Senna Danthron Bisacodyl Sodium picosulphate

Box 4.B   Management of opioid induced constipation

Ask about the patient's normal bowel habit, use of laxatives and record date of last bowel action.

Do a rectal examination if faecal impaction is suspected or if the patient reports diarrhoea or faecal incontinence (to exclude impaction with overflow).

For inpatients, record bowel motions each day in a Bowel Book.

Encourage fluids generally, and fruit juice, fruit and bran specifically.

Prescribe co-danthrusate 1 capsule nocte prophylactically.

continued

If already constipated, prescribe co-danthrusate 2 capsules nocte.

Adjust the dose every few days according to results, up to 3 capsules t.d.s.

If necessary, 'uncork' with suppositories, e.g. bisacodyl 10 mg and glycerine 4 g.

If suppositories are ineffective, administer a phosphate enema.

If the maximum dose of co-danthrusate is ineffective, reduce by half and add an osmotic laxative, e.g. lactulose 30 ml b.d.

If co-danthrusate causes abdominal cramps divide the total daily dose into smaller more frequent doses, e.g. change from co-danthrusate 2 capsules b.d. to 1 q.d.s. or change to an osmotic laxative, e.g. lactulose 20–40 ml o.d.–t.d.s.

Lactulose may be preferable to co-danthrusate in patients with a history of irritable bowel syndrome or of colic with other colonic stimulants, e.g. senna.

Sometimes it is appropriate to optimize a patient's existing bowel regimen, rather than change automatically to co-danthrusate.

If the patient prefers a liquid preparation, use co-danthrusate suspension.

Bowel obstruction

The focus here is on patients for whom available anticancer therapies have been exhausted.

Causes

- the cancer itself
- past treatment, e.g. adhesions, postradiation, ischaemic fibrosis
- associated with debility, e.g. constipation
- drugs, e.g. opioids, anticholinergics
- an unrelated benign condition, e.g. strangulated hernia
- a combination of factors.

In consequence, bowel obstruction may be

- mechanical or functional or both

- high or low or both
- single or multiple sites
- partial or complete
- transient or persistent.

Clinical features

Continuous abdominal pain associated with the underlying cancer is almost always present. Vomiting occurs in about 80% and intestinal colic in about the same proportion. Distension is variable and bowel habit ranges from absolute constipation to diarrhoea. Bowel sounds vary from absent in adynamic obstructions to hyperactive (borborygmi) in some dynamic obstructions. Tinkling bowel sounds are uncommon.

Surgical management

Surgical intervention is contra-indicated in each of the following circumstances

- previous laparotomy findings preclude the prospect of a successful intervention
- intra-abdominal carcinomatosis as evidenced by diffuse palpable intra-abdominal tumours
- massive ascites which re-accumulates rapidly after paracentesis.[41]

Surgical intervention should be considered if the following criteria are fulfilled

- an easily reversible cause seems likely, e.g. postoperative adhesions or a single discrete neoplastic obstruction
- the patient's general condition is good, i.e. he does not have widely disseminated disease and has been independent and active
- the patient is willing to undergo surgery.

Medical management

In patients in whom an operative approach is contra-indicated, it is generally possible to relieve symptoms adequately with drugs. A nasogastric tube and IV fluids are rarely necessary.

Eliminate pain and colic

- for constant background pain, administer diamorphine/morphine by continuous SC infusion using a portable syringe driver
- if the patient is experiencing colic:
  do not use a prokinetic drug
  discontinue bulk forming, osmotic and stimulant laxatives
- if colic persists despite SC diamorphine/morphine, prescribe SC hyoscine butylbromide 60–120 mg/24 h in addition.

Eliminate nausea and reduce vomiting to once or twice a day

The choice of anti-emetic depends on whether the patient is experiencing colic. If yes, hyoscine butylbromide will have been started already. If no, the following sequence can be followed

- if passing flatus, a *trial* of SC metoclopramide 60–120 mg/24 h helps to determine whether the obstruction is more functional than mechanical
- if not helpful, prescribe SC cyclizine 100–150 mg/24 h
- if cyclizine fails, SC hyoscine butylbromide 60–120 mg/24 h should be tried because of its antisecretory properties
- SC octreotide 300–600 mcg/24 h may be used instead; this expensive somatostatin analogue has similar intestinal effects to hyoscine butyl-bromide but no anticholinergic effects; about two thirds of patients benefit
- if there is persistent nausea (generally caused by toxic factors), add haloperidol 5–10 mg/24 h
- SC levomepromazine 6.25–25 mg/24 h can be tried instead, alone or in combination with hyoscine butylbromide
- a venting gastrostomy is rarely needed.

Because bowel distension causes the release of 5HT/serotonin from entero-chromaffin cells in the bowel, some patients will benefit from a $5HT_3$ receptor antagonist.

Corticosteroids benefit only a few patients. Benefit from corticosteroids must be differentiated from spontaneous remission – seen in about one third of cancer patients with partial obstruction.

Relieve associated constipation

A phosphate enema should be given if constipation is a likely causal factor and a faecal softener prescribed, i.e. docusate tablets 100–200 mg b.d. If the small bowel only is affected, a colonic stimulant laxative can be used.

General

Inoperable patients managed by drug therapy should be encouraged to drink and eat small amounts of their favourite beverages and food. Some patients find that they can manage food best in the morning.

The use of anticholinergic drugs and diminished fluid intake often result in a dry mouth and thirst. These symptoms are generally relieved by conscientious mouth care. A few ml of fluid every 30 minutes, possibly administered as a small ice cube, often brings relief. IV hydration is rarely needed.

Ascites

Ascites may cause several symptoms of differing intensity (Table 4.5).

Table 4.5   Clinical features of ascites

Abdominal distension	Acid reflux
Abdominal discomfort/pain	Nausea and vomiting
Inability to sit upright	Leg oedema
Early satiety	Dyspnoea
Dyspepsia	

Pathogenesis

- generally associated with peritoneal metastases
- subphrenic lymphatics become blocked by tumour infiltration
- increased peritoneal permeability
- hyperaldosteronism, possibly secondary to reduced extracellular blood volume, causes sodium retention and further feeds the ascitic process
- liver metastases leading to hypo-albuminaemia and, sometimes, portal hypertension.

Management

Diuretics

Spironolactone is the key to success because it antagonizes aldosterone (Table 4.6). Two thirds of patients are controlled on spironolactone 300 mg o.d. or less.

Table 4.6　Diuretic treatment of malignant ascites

	Spironolactone	Loop diuretic	
		Bumetanide or Furosemide	
Day 1	100–200 mg o.d.	–	–
Day 7	200–300 mg o.d.	1 mg	40 mg
Day 14	200 mg b.d.	2 mg	80 mg

The dose of the loop diuretic should be reduced once a satisfactory result is achieved.

Failure with diuretic therapy generally relates to

- gastric intolerance (spironolactone)
- therapeutic impatience
- too small a dose of spironolactone
- failure to use concomitant loop diuretic in resistant cases.

Paracentesis

Paracentesis is used for a distressed patient with a tense painful abdomen. Remove as much fluid as possible using an IV cannula or suprapubic catheter. Repeat if diuretics do not prevent re-accumulation.

Peritoneovenous shunt

This is an option in a patient who is relatively well but cannot tolerate diuretic therapy. It is not often appropriate.

Respiratory symptoms

Dyspnoea

All advanced cancer 50%; lung cancer 70%. Incidence increases in the final weeks.

Dyspnoea is usually associated with *tachypnoea*. If the resting respiratory rate is 30–35/min, activity or additional anxiety may increase this to 50–60/min.

Causes

Various respiratory drives predispose to dyspnoea (Table 4.7).

Table 4.7   Respiratory drives

Wakefulness	Lung deflation
Anxiety, fear	Acidosis
Anger, rage	Hypercapnia
Pyrexia	Hypoxia
Lung distortion	

Some patients with effort dyspnoea experience respiratory panic attacks. These are often brought on by activity, e.g. going upstairs. During these attacks the patient is convinced he is going to die:

dyspnoea + lack of understanding + fear → increased anxiety → increased respiratory rate → increased dyspnoea etc.

Dyspnoea is often caused by multiple factors (Table 4.8). A dyspnoeic patient is often an anxious patient, particularly if dyspnoeic at rest.

Management

Explanation

Respond to or anticipate patient's questions, e.g. 'Will I choke to death?', 'Will I suffocate?', 'Will I stop breathing if I go to sleep?'

Emphasize, 'Becoming breathless in itself is not dangerous'.

Table 4.8   Causes of dyspnoea in advanced cancer

Caused by cancer	Related to cancer and/or debility
Effusion(s)	Anaemia
Obstruction of a main bronchus	Atelectasis
Replacement of lung by cancer	Pulmonary embolism
Lymphangitis carcinomatosa	Pneumonia
Mediastinal obstruction	Empyema
Pericardial effusion	Weakness
Massive ascites	
Abdominal distension	
Cachexia	*Concurrent causes*
	COPD
Caused by treatment	Asthma
	Heart failure
Pneumonectomy	Acidosis
Radiation induced fibrosis	
Chemotherapy	
bleomycin	
doxorubicin	

Respiratory panic attacks

● prophylactic education about and practice in breathing control

● a calming presence.

Treat reversible causes (Table 4.9)

Nondrug measures

● a calming presence

● cool draught

● breathing exercises

● relaxation therapy.

Modify way of life

● sit to wash/shave

Table 4.9   Specific treatment of dyspnoea in advanced cancer

Cause	Treatment
Respiratory infection	Antibiotic Expectorant Physiotherapy
COPD/asthma	Bronchodilators Corticosteroids Physiotherapy
Hypoxia	Trial of oxygen
Bronchial obstruction/lung collapse ⎫ Mediastinal obstruction ⎬	Corticosteroids Radiotherapy LASER therapy Stent
Lymphangitis carcinomatosa	Corticosteroids
Pleural effusion	Aspiration Pleuradesis
Ascites	Diuretics Paracentesis
Pericardial effusion	Paracentesis Corticosteroids
Anaemia	Blood transfusion
Cardiac failure	Diuretics ACE inhibitors
Pulmonary embolism	Anticoagulants (?)

- help with housework
- bed downstairs
- bed rest.

Drugs for dyspnoea

- morphine; the aim is to ease the sensation of dyspnoea:
    if on morphine for pain, increase the dose by 50%
    if not on oral morphine, 5–6 mg q4h is a good starting dose
    (Note: by *nebulizer*, morphine is no better than saline[42])

- diazepam if the patient is very anxious:
  5–10 mg stat and 5–20 mg nocte
  in the very elderly, 2–5 mg
  reduce dose after several days if drowsy

- oxygen 4 l/min via nasal prongs if dyspnoeic at rest.

Special situations

Acute tracheal compression/massive haemorrhage into trachea

This is a very rare palliative care emergency

- IV diazepam/midazolam until patient unconscious (5–20 mg)
- PR diazepam or IM midazolam 20 mg, if IV administration not possible
- continuous company.

Noisy tachypnoea in the moribund

Although the patient is not aware, the family and other patients become distressed. Consider slowing the respiratory rate down to 10–15/min with IV diamorphine/morphine. It may be necessary to give double or treble the previously satisfactory analgesic dose to contain this form of tachypnoea. If there is associated heaving of the shoulders and chest, midazolam should be given as well, e.g. 10 mg SC stat and hourly as needed.

Cough

Causes

These include

- intrathoracic cancer
- chest infection
- chronic bronchitis
- smoking.

Types of cough

- wet cough and patient able to cough effectively
- wet cough but patient too weak to cough effectively
- dry cough, i.e. nonproductive of sputum.

Management

Treat reversible causes (Table 4.10)

Table 4.10   Reversible causes of cough

Cause	Treatment
Cigarettes	Stop smoking
Postnasal drip	Antihistamine
Respiratory infection	Antibiotic (if purulent sputum) Expectorant Physiotherapy
COPD/asthma	Bronchodilator Corticosteroid Physiotherapy
Cardiac failure	Diuretic ACE inhibitor
Drug induced (e.g. ACE inhibitor)	Stop or change drug
Oesophageal reflux	Patient should sleep semi-upright Stop or reduce dose of drug causing a reduction of lower oesophageal sphincter tone Metoclopramide, cisapride to increase lower oesophageal spincter tone
Aspiration of saliva	Anticholinergic to reduce saliva
Malignant obstruction	Corticosteroids Radiation therapy Chemotherapy

Nondrug measures

● advise how to cough effectively; it is impossible to cough effectively lying on your back

● postural drainage

● physiotherapy.

Mucolytics/expectorants

- saline 2–5% in nebulizer (the only mucolytic used at Sobell House)
- chemical inhalations:
  compound benzoin tincture (Friar's balsam)
  carbol
  menthol and eucalyptus
- irritant mucolytics:
  guaiphenesin
  ipecacuanha
  potassium iodide
- chemical mucolytics:
  acetylcysteine
  carbocysteine.

Antitussives

- simple linctus
- codeine linctus
- strong opioid, e.g. morphine, methadone.

Hiccup

Definition

Hiccup is a pathological respiratory reflex characterized by spasm of the diaphragm, resulting in sudden inspiration and associated with closure of the vocal cords.

Causes

There are innumerable potential causes of hiccup. In advanced cancer, the following account for most cases

- gastric distension
- diaphragmatic irritation
- phrenic nerve irritation
- toxicity:
  uraemia
  infection

- CNS tumour.

Of these, gastric distension probably accounts for 95% of cases.

Acute management options

Pharyngeal stimulation (triggers a 'gating' mechanism)

- drinking from 'wrong' side of a cup *or* cold key down back of neck (acts via hyperextension of neck)
- granulated sugar (two heaped teaspoons) *or* liqueur (two glasses) rapidly ingested
- pulling tongue out of mouth forcibly
- nebulized saline (2 ml 0.9% over 5 minutes).[43]

Massage of the junction between hard and soft palate with a cotton bob is also an effective gating mechanism.

Reduce gastric distension

- peppermint water facilitates belching by relaxing the lower oesophageal sphincter (an old-fashioned remedy)
- antiflatulent, e.g. Asilone 10 ml
- metoclopramide 10 mg (tightens the lower oesophageal sphincter and hastens gastric emptying).

Peppermint water and metoclopramide should not be used concurrently.

Elevation of pCO_2

This inhibits processing of the hiccup reflex in the brain stem

- rebreathing from a paper bag
- breath holding.

Muscle relaxant

- baclofen 10 mg PO
- nifedipine 10 mg PO
- midazolam 5–10 mg IV.

Central suppression of hiccup reflex

- haloperidol 5 mg PO or IV if no response
- chlorpromazine 10–25 mg PO or IV if no response.

Maintenance treatment

Gastric distension

- antiflatulent, e.g. Asilone 10 ml qds and/or
- metoclopramide 10 mg q.d.s.

Diaphragmatic irritation or other cause

- baclofen 5–10 mg b.d.–20 mg q8h
- nifedipine 10–20 mg q8h, occasionally more[44]
- haloperidol 5–10 mg nocte
- midazolam 10–60 mg/24 h by SC infusion if all else fails.

Urinary symptoms

Useful definitions

Frequency	Passage of urine seven or more times during the day and twice or more at night.
Urgency	A strong and sudden desire to void.
Urge incontinence	The involuntary loss of urine associated with a strong desire to void.
Detrusor instability	Detrusor contracts uninhibitedly and causes: diurnal frequency increasing severity nocturnal frequency urgency urge incontinence (Detrusor instability is the second most common cause of urinary incontinence in women.)
Stress incontinence	The involuntary loss of urine associated with coughing, sneezing, laughing and lifting.

continued

Genuine stress incontinence (Urethral sphincter incompetence)	The involuntary loss of urine when the intravesical pressure exceeds maximum urethral pressure in the *absence of detrusor activity*. The fault always lies in the sphincter mechanisms of the bladder, and is associated with multiparity, postmenopause and posthysterectomy.
	One or more of the following features will be present:
	descent of urethrovesical junction outside intra-abdominal zone of pressure
	decrease in urethral pressure due to loss of urethral wall elasticity and contractility
	short functional length of the urethra.
	(Urethral sphincter incompetence is the most common cause of urinary incontinence in women.)
Dysuria	Pain during and/or after micturition. Often urethral in origin (a burning sensation) but may be caused by bladder spasm (intense suprapubic and urethral pain), or both.

Urinary bladder innervation

*'You **pee** with your **parasympathetics**.
You **stop** with your **sympathetics**.'*

The sphincter relaxes when the detrusor (bladder muscle) contracts, and vice versa (Table 4.11). Thus, anticholinergic (antimuscarinic) drugs not only cause contraction of the bladder neck sphincter but also relax the detrusor.

Detrusor sensitivity is

- increased by prostaglandins

- decreased by COX inhibitors i.e. NSAIDs.

The urethral sphincter is an additional voluntary mechanism innervated by the pudendal nerve (S2–4).

The urethra, derived embryologically from the urogenital sinus, is sensitive in the female to oestrogen and progesterone. Postmenopausal urge incontinence and frequency is sometimes helped by the prescription of an oestrogen, either topically or orally. Oestrogens do not improve stress incontinence.

Table 4.11   Autonomic innervation of urinary bladder

		Effect on	
Innervation	Mediator	Sphincter	Vault
Sympathetic (T10–12, L1)	Norepinephrine	Contracts (α)	Relaxes (β)
Parasympathetic (S2–4)	Acetylcholine	Relaxes	Contracts

Table 4.12   Morphine and the urinary tract

Bladder sensation decreased
Sphincter tone *increased*
Detrusor tone *increased*
Ureteric tone and amplitude of contractions increased

Morphine and other opioids have several effects on bladder function (Table 4.12). These are generally asymptomatic. Occasionally hesitancy or retention occurs.

Causes

The most common urinary symptoms in advanced cancer are

- frequency and urgency
- incontinence
- hesitancy and retention
- bladder spasms.

Causes to be considered are listed in Tables 4.13–4.15. As in other areas of symptom management, careful evaluation is fundamental. Rectal examination to exclude faecal impaction may be necessary in debilitated/moribund patients, particularly if there is associated delirium.

Table 4.13   Causes of urgency and incontinence

Caused by cancer	Related to cancer and/or debility
Pain	Infective cystitis
Hypercalcaemia (causes polyuria)	
Intravesical ⎱ mechanical	*Concurrent causes*
Extravesical ⎰ irritation	Idiopathic detrusor instability
Bladder spasms	Central neurological disease
Sacral plexopathy	poststroke
	multiple sclerosis
Caused by treatment	dementia
	Uraemia ⎫
Radiation cystitis	Diabetes mellitus ⎬ cause polyuria
Cyclophosphamide cystitis	Diabetes insipidus ⎭
Drugs	
diuretics	
opioids	

Table 4.14   Causes of hesitancy and retention

Caused by cancer	Related to cancer and/or debility
Malignant enlargement of prostate	Loaded rectum
Infiltration of bladder neck	Inability to stand to micturate
Presacral plexopathy	Generalized weakness
Spinal cord compression	
	Concurrent causes
Caused by treatment	Benign enlargement of prostate
Anticholinergic drugs (see p.127)	
Morphine (occasionally)	
Spinal analgesia (particularly with bupivacaine)	
Intrathecal nerve block	

Table 4.15   Causes of bladder spasms

Caused by cancer	Related to cancer and/or debility
Intravesical ⎱ irritation	Anxiety
Extravesical ⎰	Infective cystitis
	Indwelling catheter
Caused by treatment	mechanical irritation by catheter balloon
	catheter sludging with partial retention
Radiation fibrosis	

Management

Management depends on the cause and commonly comprises both nondrug and drug approaches. The detection and treatment of urinary infection is obviously important if causing dysuria, urgency and frequency. 'Bladder drill' (e.g. voiding every 2 h by the clock) may be helpful in someone with urge incontinence.

Drugs of choice

Urgency

- oxybutynin 2.5–5 mg b.d.–q.d.s.
- amitriptyline 25–50 mg nocte
- propantheline 15 mg b.d.–t.d.s.

Treatment may be limited by anticholinergic effects.

Hesitancy

- indoramin 20 mg nocte–b.d., a selective α-1 adrenoceptor antagonist (maximum dose 100 mg/24 h)
- bethanechol 10–30 mg b.d.–q.d.s., a cholinergic drug.

Bladder spasm

- if catheterized, change catheter or reduce volume of balloon
- if urinary infection:
  no catheter – treat with systemic antibiotic
  catheter – treat with bladder washouts and/or urinary antiseptics, e.g. methenamine hippurate 1 g b.d.
- anticholinergic drug (as for urgency)
- flavoxate 200–400 mg t.d.s.–q.d.s. (a weak detrusor relaxant) if anticholinergic drugs cause unacceptable adverse effects.

Discoloured urine

There are many causes of discoloured urine. The patient and his family fear that it is evidence of further deterioration. If the urine is red, it is assumed to be haematuria.

Diet

- rhubarb→*red*
- beetroot→red

Drugs

- doxorubicin→*red*
- danthron (in co-danthramer and co-danthrusate)→*red/green/blue*
- nefopam→*pink*
- phenolphthalein→*pink* (in alkaline urine); present in several proprietary laxatives, e.g. Agarol
- phenazopyridine→*yellow/orange*
- methylene blue→*blue*; present in certain proprietary urinary antiseptic mixtures, e.g. Urised in the USA.

Infection

Pseudomonas aeruginosa (pyocyanin)→*blue* (in alkaline urine).

Other symptoms

Hypercalcaemia

Hypercalcaemia may cause many nonspecific symptoms, e.g. dry mouth, thirst, anorexia, nausea and vomiting, constipation, frequency (polyuria), lethargy, weakness, depression.

Incidence

All malignant disease 10–20%. Breast, squamous lung and genito-urinary cancers and myeloma 20–40%. Uncommon in prostate, small cell lung, gastric and large bowel cancers.

Diagnosis is based on a high level of clinical suspicion and confirmed by blood tests, 'correcting' for hypo-albuminaemia.

Management

Stop and think! Are you justified in treating a potentially fatal complication in a moribund patient?

The following together comprise a set of indications for treating hyper-calcaemia

- corrected plasma calcium concentration of > 2.8 mmol/l
- severe symptoms attributable to hypercalcaemia
- first episode or long interval since previous one
- previous good quality of life (in patient's opinion)
- medical judgement that measures will achieve a durable effect (based on the results of previous treatment)
- patient willing to undergo IV therapy and requisite blood tests.

Bisphosphonates

IV rehydration with normal saline, e.g. 3 l/24 h, and IV bisphosphonate, e.g. pamidronate 30–45 mg or clodronate 1500 mg by infusion in saline over 2–8 h

- bisphosphonates act by inhibiting osteoclasts
- maximum effect 5–7 days with pamidronate; 3–5 days with clodronate
- repeat after 4–7 days if initial poor response
- effect generally lasts 3+ weeks with pamidronate; less with clodronate.

Spinal cord compression

Incidence

Spinal cord compression occurs in 3% of patients with advanced cancer. Cancers of the breast and bronchus and lymphoma account for 40%. Most occur in the thorax. There is compression at more than one level in 20%.

Below the level of L2 vertebra, compression is of the cauda equina, i.e. peripheral nerves only are involved, and not the spinal cord.

Presentation

- pain   > 90%

- weakness   > 75%
- sensory level   > 50%
- sphincter dysfunction   > 40%.

The patient may be unaware of sensory loss until examined, particularly if this is confined to the sacrum or perineum.

Pain generally predates other symptoms and signs of cord compression by weeks or months. Pain may be caused by

- vertebral metastasis
- root compression
- compression of the long tracts of the spinal cord (funicular pain).

Radicular and funicular pains are often exacerbated by neck flexion or straight leg raising, and by coughing, sneezing or straining. Funicular pain is generally less sharp than radicular pain, has a more diffuse distribution (like a cuff or garter around thighs, knees or calves) and is sometimes described as a cold unpleasant sensation.

Diagnosis

- history and clinical findings
- a plain radiograph shows vertebral metastasis collapse at the appropriate level in 80%
- a bone scan does not often yield additional information
- MRI is the investigation of choice
- CT with myelography may be helpful if MRI is not available.

Management

- dexamethasone; the dose used varies greatly. One regimen is 12 mg PO stat and then 16–32 mg o.d. for 1 week; after which it is reduced/stopped over the next 2–3 weeks
- radiation therapy concurrently

- consider decompressive surgery if:
    diagnosis in doubt
    solitary vertebral metastasis
    deterioration despite radiotherapy and high dose dexamethasone.

If the cord compression is of rapid onset (1–2 days), the most likely cause is infarction of the spinal cord as a consequence of spinal artery thrombosis secondary to compression/distortion by malignant disease. This does not respond to treatment.

Lymphoedema

Definition

Lymphoedema is excessive interstitial fluid with a high protein content associated with chronic inflammation and fibrosis.

Lymphoedema can occur in any part of the body, generally a limb with or without adjacent trunk involvement. It is progressive and, if left untreated, becomes a gross and debilitating condition. Acute inflammation (whether infective or not) and trauma cause a rapid increase in swelling.

Causes

Lymphoedema may be

- primary, e.g. congenital, hereditary (Milroy's disease), sporadic
- secondary, e.g. cancer and anticancer treatments, infections, trauma.

In the UK, cancer and anticancer treatments account for most cases of secondary lymphoedema, i.e.

- axillary or groin surgery
- postoperative infection
- radiotherapy
- axillary, groin or intrapelvic recurrence.

Clinical features

- a swollen limb which feels tight and does not resolve with elevation
- if acute, will pit on pressure; when chronic, less or no pitting

- impaired limb mobility and function

- pain related to tissue swelling and/or shoulder strain. May be concurrent neuropathic pain if there is recurrence in the axilla

- psychological distress because of altered body image, unsightliness and inability to wear short sleeved garments or shoes.

Management

Because lymphoedema cannot be cured, management focuses on maximizing improvement and long term control. The earlier treatment is started the easier it is to achieve a good result. Treatment is of three types

- standard

- intensive

- palliative.

The choice of treatment depends on

- whether there is local recurrence of cancer

- the patient's general physical condition

- the state of the swollen limb (Table 4.16).

Comments here will be limited to palliative treatment.

Table 4.16   Criteria for and aims of lymphoedema management

Therapy	Indications	Aims
Standard	Uncomplicated lymphoedema	Long term control of swelling

Intensive	Complicated
	    awkwardly shaped limb,
	      e.g. deep skin folds
	    digit swelling
	    severe trunk swelling
		Improve skin condition
		Reduce volume
		Reshape limb
		Disrupt fibrosis
		Restore function and mobility

Palliative	Local recurrence of cancer
	causing or exacerbating
	lymphoedema
		Prevent or alleviate
		  infection
		  pain
		  increasing swelling
		  lymphorrhoea
		Maintain function and mobility

Skin care

Wash and moisturize daily, e.g. with aqueous cream. This is often best done at bedtime. Give advice about avoiding trauma, thereby reducing the likelihood of infection.

Massage

Simple skin-moving massage of the affected limb and adjacent trunk b.d. This stimulates skin lymphatics to contract, thereby increasing superficial lymphatic drainage. *Areas affected by cancer should not be massaged.* If appropriate, relatives can be taught to massage the skin.

Compression

International standard graduation compression garments class 1–3 or Shaped Tubigrip or light support bandaging, e.g. Setopress, applied daily with soft padding.

Exercise

Encourage normal use or gentle active or passive movements. If flaccid, use a broad arm sling when standing. Support the heavy limb when resting.

Patients must wear compression bandaging or a containment garment during exercise. The compression enhances the effect of muscle contraction on lymph flow and surface friction stimulates contractions in the superficial lymphatics.

Other

- a diuretic should be used if the swelling developed or worsened after the prescription of a NSAID or a corticosteroid, or if there is a venous component. Otherwise, do *not* prescribe because it will have no effect on protein-rich oedema.

- a pneumatic compression pump is helpful in shifting *venous* oedema. Its use may speed up the rate of initial improvement in patients with combined lymphovenous oedema.

Pruritus

Causes

- dry flaky skin (xerosis)
- wet macerated skin

- skin disease, e.g. contact dermatitis, scabies
- drug reaction
- cholestatic jaundice
- renal failure
- paraneoplastic, particularly in Hodgkin's lymphoma (15%)
- diabetes – usually localized and related to candidiasis
- psychiatric.

Management

A dry skin is almost always present in patients with advanced cancer who experience pruritus, even when there is a definite endogenous cause. Measures to correct skin dryness should precede specific measures, or go hand in hand with them.

Pruritus in renal failure is often more difficult to treat. It is associated with an increase in dermal mast cells and divalent ions (magnesium and calcium). In patients with hypercalcaemia associated with secondary hyperparathyroidism, correction of hypercalcaemia leads to the rapid relief of pruritus.

General measures

- discourage scratching; keep nails cut short; allow gentle rubbing
- discontinue use of soap
- use emulsifying ointment or aqueous cream as a soap substitute, or add Oilatum to bath water
- avoid hot, long baths
- dry skin gently by patting with soft towel
- avoid overheating and sweating.

Topical measures for worst affected areas

- aqueous cream (± 1% menthol) applied to skin after bath and each evening
- crotamiton (Eurax) cream b.d.–t.d.s. has both mild antipruritic and anti-scabetic properties. It is rarely necessary
- oily calamine lotion as required (contains 0.5% phenol as an antipruritic)

- clioquinol (Vioform)-hydrocortisone cream if inflamed b.d.–t.d.s.

Drugs

Drugs are of little benefit if used without skin care. Most patients with advanced cancer and pruritus never need an antihistamine if given appropriate skin care.

Cholestyramine (an anion exchange resin which binds bile acids) is not recommended in obstructive jaundice. It is not often effective, causes diarrhoea and is unpalatable. Stenting of the common bile duct is, of course, the preferred option. If not feasible, an androgen eases pruritus in 5–10 days, e.g. stanozolol 5–10 mg o.d.

In both obstructive jaundice and renal failure, $5HT_3$ receptor antagonists in standard anti-emetic doses will relieve pruritus within hours.[45]

Secondary mental disorders

Definition

These are mental disorders which are secondary to organic disease or related to chemical substances (drugs, alcohol) or both (synonym: organic mental disorders).

Classification

Secondary mental disorders are classified mainly on the basis of their key features (Table 4.17).

Table 4.17   Secondary mental disorders

Delirium	Delusional disorder
Dementia	Personality disorder
Amnestic disorder	Intoxication
Anxiety disorder	Withdrawal state
Mood disorder	Psychosis
Hallucinosis	

All secondary mental disorders may be seen in patients with advanced cancer.

Delirium (synonyms: acute brain syndrome, acute confusional state), dementia (synonym: chronic brain syndrome) and secondary amnestic disorder are all characterized by cognitive impairment. The word confusion is often used of all three conditions. Note that

● sometimes dementia is compounded by delirium

● dementia is not usually associated with drowsiness

● some patients with cancer appear to develop dementia rapidly – and this may cause difficulty in diagnosis (Table 4.18).

Table 4.18   Comparison of global cognitive impairment disorders

Delirium		Dementia
Acute		Chronic
Often remitting and reversible		Usually progressive and irreversible
Mental clouding (information not taken in)		Brain damage (information not retained)
+	Poor concentration	+
+	Impaired short term memory	+
+	Disorientation	+
+	Living in the past	+
+	Misinterpretations	+
++	Hallucinations	+
+	Delusions	+
Speech rambling and incoherent		Speech stereotyped and limited
Often diurnal variation		Constant (in later stages)
Often aware and anxious		Unaware and unconcerned (in later stages)

Patients with cognitive impairment disorders have identifiable cognitive defects if tested formally using, for example, the Mini-Mental State Examination.

Patients manifesting the following are sometimes misdiagnosed as confused

● not taking in what is said:

    deaf
    anxious
    too ill to concentrate

- muddled speech:
  poor concentration
  nominal dysphasia.

It is also important to identify hypnagogic (when going to sleep) and hypnopompic (when waking up) hallucinations as these are normal phenomena, although more common in ill patients receiving sedative drugs.

Causes

Dementia is usually caused by Alzheimer's disease or cerebral atherosclerosis; occasionally it may be paraneoplastic. The causes of other secondary mental disorders are

- drugs

- biochemical derangement

- organ failure

- brain tumours

- paraneoplastic.

Delirium

Delirium (acute confusional state) is associated with mental clouding. This leads to a disturbance of comprehension and bewilderment. Manifestations include

- poor concentration

- impairment of short term memory

- disorientation

- misinterpretations

- paranoid ideas

- hallucinations

- rambling incoherent speech

- restlessness

- noisy/aggressive behaviour.

Table 4.19   Precipitating factors for delirium in advanced cancer

Change of environment	Pain
Unfamiliar excessive stimuli	Constipation
too hot	Urinary retention
too cold	
wet bed	Infection
crumbs in bed	Dehydration
creases in sheets	
	Withdrawal state
Anxiety	alcohol
	nicotine
Depression	psychotropic drugs
Fatigue	Vitamin deficiency

There may be associated drowsiness. Psychomotor activity may be increased or decreased. Increased activity may be associated with overactivity of the autonomic nervous system, i.e. facial flushing, dilated pupils, injected conjunctivae, tachycardia and sweating. Delirium is precipitated or exacerbated by many factors (Table 4.19).

Management

Hallucinations, nightmares and misinterpretations represent a failure in the patient's coping mechanisms, and reflect fears and anxieties. Their content should be explored with the patient.

Explanation

- stress to both the patient and the relatives that the patient is not going mad, and there is a physical cause
- stress that there are generally lucid intervals
- continue to treat the patient with courtesy and respect.

General measures

- restraints should never be used
- bed rails should be avoided – they can be dangerous
- patient should be allowed to walk about accompanied
- allay fear and suspicion, and reduce misinterpretations by:

use of night light
not changing the position of the patient's bed
explaining every procedure and event in detail
the presence of a family member or close friend.

Drugs

Generally use drugs only if symptoms are marked, persistent and cause distress to the patient and/or family. Review sooner rather than later if a sedative drug is prescribed because symptoms may be exacerbated.

Consider

- reduction in medication

- oxygen if cyanosed

- dexamethasone if cerebral tumour (*see* p.120)

- haloperidol 1.5–5 mg PO or SC if agitated, hallucinating or paranoid.

The initial dose of haloperidol depends on previous medication, weight, age and severity of symptoms. Subsequent doses depend on the initial response; o.d.–b.d. maintenance doses are generally adequate.

Terminal distress

This is often associated with delirium and may need haloperidol 10–30 mg/24 h and/or midazolam 10–60 mg/24 h by continuous SC infusion to control it.

Levomepromazine 25–50 mg stat and 50–200 mg/24 h should be substituted for haloperidol if the patient remains agitated despite the combined use of haloperidol and midazolam. Alternatively SC phenobarbital 100–200 mg stat and 800–1600 mg/24 h may need to be used instead of both haloperidol and midazolam.

Drug profiles

Corticosteroids

Corticosteroids are used for many reasons in advanced cancer (Table 4.20). Inclusion in the table does *not* mean that a corticosteroid is necessarily the treatment of choice in that situation.

Table 4.20   Indications for corticosteroids in advanced cancer

Specific

Spinal cord compression

Nerve compression

Dyspnoea
   pneumonitis (after radiotherapy)
   lymphangitis carcinomatosa
   tracheal compression/stridor

Superior vena caval obstruction

Pericardial effusion

Haemoptysis

Obstruction of hollow viscus
   bronchus
   ureter
   [bowel]

Hypercalcaemia (in corticosteroid responsive tumours, e.g. lymphoma, myeloma)

Radiation induced inflammation

Leuco-erythroblastic anaemia

Rectal discharge (give PR)

Sweating

Pain relief

Raised intracranial pressure

Nerve compression

Spinal cord compression

Metastatic arthralgia

[Bone pain]

Hormone therapy

Replacement

Anticancer

General

To improve appetite

To enhance sense of wellbeing

To improve strength

At Sobell House, dexamethasone is the corticosteroid of choice. It is generally given in a single daily dose. Dexamethasone has a duration of effect of 36–54 h, compared with 18–36 h for prednisolone.

Dexamethasone is seven times more potent than prednisolone. Thus, 2 mg of dexamethasone is approximately equivalent to 15 mg of prednisolone. Dexamethasone is available in 0.5 mg and 2 mg tablets, and also as an injection. Prednisolone is available in a range of tablets from 1–25 mg.

The initial daily dose varies according to indication and fashion, ranging from dexamethasone 2–4 mg (prednisolone 15–30 mg) for anorexia to 16–32 mg for spinal cord compression. A dose of 8–16 mg is generally used for raised intracranial pressure.

Oral candidiasis and ankle oedema are common adverse effects. Moonfacing, hyperphagia, weight gain, myopathy or diabetes mellitus may necessitate dose reduction and, sometimes, cessation of treatment.

Agitation, insomnia or a more florid psychiatric disturbance may be precipitated by corticosteroids – either when commencing or stopping treatment.

Apart from hydrocortisone, corticosteroids should generally be given in a single daily dose in the morning to ease compliance and to prevent insomnia. Even so, temazepam or diazepam at bedtime is sometimes needed to counter insomnia or agitation.

Antacids

An antacid is a chemical substance taken by mouth to neutralize gastric acid. Generic antacids include

- sodium bicarbonate
- magnesium salts (cause diarrhoea)
- aluminium hydroxide (causes constipation)
- hydrotalcite (i.e. magnesium aluminium carbonate)
- calcium carbonate.

Points to remember

Some antacids contain significant amounts of sodium. This may be important in patients with hypertension or cardiac failure. Liquid Gaviscon (see p.121) and magnesium trisilicate mixture both contain > 6 mmol/10 ml compared with 0.1 mmol/10 ml in Asilone. The regular use of sodium bicarbonate may cause sodium loading and metabolic alkalosis.

Aluminium hydroxide binds dietary phosphate. It is of benefit in patients with hyperphosphataemia in renal failure. The long term complications of phosphate depletion and osteomalacia are not generally an issue in advanced cancer.

Hydrotalcite binds bile salts and is therefore of specific benefit in patients with bile salt reflux, e.g. after certain forms of gastroduodenal surgery.

The regular use of calcium carbonate may cause hypercalcaemia, particularly if taken with sodium bicarbonate.

Preparations

Proprietary preparations usually contain a mixture of magnesium and aluminium so as to neutralize any effect on bowel habit. They may also contain sodium bicarbonate.

Some antacids contain additional substances

- activated dimeticone is an antifoaming agent present in Asilone, a proprietary antacid. By facilitating belching, dimeticone eases flatulence, distension and postprandial gastric distension pain

- alginic acid (in Gaviscon) prevents oesophageal reflux pain by forming an inert low density raft on the top of the acid stomach contents. Gaviscon needs both *acid* and *air bubbles* to produce the raft. It may be less effective if used with an H₂ receptor antagonist (reduces acid) and/or antiflatulent (reduces air bubbles)

- oxetacaine (in Mucaine) eases reflux pain by coating and anaesthetizing damaged oesophageal mucosa.

Diazepam

Properties and uses

- anxiolytic
- night sedative
- muscle relaxant
- anticonvulsant.

Diazepam is sometimes used as a secondary anti-emetic in patients receiving chemotherapy.

Limitations

- daytime drowsiness
- muscular flaccidity
- postural hypotension.

General comments

- plasma halflife 20–100 h; generally given once a day at *bedtime*. If patient does not sleep at night, daytime drowsiness more likely
- patients occasionally react paradoxically, i.e. become more distressed; if this happens, change to haloperidol or chlorpromazine
- diazepam acts faster PO or PR than IM because the standard preparation is oil-based; IV may cause thrombophlebitis
- if available, use diazepam oil-in-water emulsion (Diazemuls) for IV injection; this is less irritant.

Therapeutic guidelines

Initial dose depends on

- patient's previous experience of diazepam and other benzodiazepines
- intensity of distress
- urgency of relief.

The following doses are a guide

- 2 mg is useful and safe in the elderly
- 5 mg is the typical initial dose
- 10 mg may be necessary in severe distress, particularly in younger patients.

Repeat *hourly* until the desired effect is achieved, and then decide on an appropriate maintenance regimen.

Rectal diazepam is useful in a crisis or if the patient is moribund

- suppositories 10 mg
- rectal solution 5–10 mg in 2.5 ml

● parenteral formulation inserted through a cannula.

Lorazepam 1 mg tablets can be given SL as an alternative; this is equivalent to diazepam 10 mg.

Patterns of use

● as needed is the best initial way in the elderly, and for acute (possibly transient) episodes of severe anxiety

● regularly at bedtime is best for those with persistent anxiety – to be used as an adjunct to psychological measures; also if used for muscle spasm or general stiffness

● more than daily (e.g. 1000/1400, 2200 h or 1000, 1800, 2200 h) in agitated moribund patients to reduce the number of hours the patient is awake and distressed.

Midazolam

The main advantage of midazolam is that it is water-soluble and is miscible with most of the drugs commonly given by continuous SC infusion. It is also easier for IV injection.

Properties and uses

● anaesthetic induction agent

● sedative for minor procedures

● sedative for terminal agitation

● anticonvulsant.

Midazolam versus diazepam

In single doses

● for sedation, midazolam is three times as potent

● as an anticonvulsant, midazolam is twice as potent.

With multiple doses, diazepam will gain in potency because of its prolonged plasma halflife, i.e. 20–100 h versus 1–4 h for midazolam (but about 10 h when given by infusion).

Patterns of use

Typical doses for midazolam are shown in Table 4.21.

Table 4.21   Dose recommendations for SC midazolam

Indication	Stat dose	Initial infusion rate/24 h	Common range
Muscle stiffness Multifocal myoclonus	5 mg	10 mg	10–30 mg
Terminal agitation Anticonvulsant	10 mg	30 mg	30–60 mg

In terminal agitation, if the patient is not settled on 30 mg/24 h, introduce a neuroleptic drug before increasing the dose of midazolam further.

Haloperidol

Properties and uses

- anti-emetic
- antipsychotic
- anxiolytic.

Limitations

- anticholinergic effects
- extrapyramidal reactions
- drowsiness.

General comments

- plasma halflife 12–20 h; can generally be given o. d.
- in higher doses (> 5 mg) has a sedative effect, and may substitute satisfactorily for a night sedative

- extrapyramidal reactions more likely at daily doses of > 5 mg. Because these occur inconsistently, an antiparkinsonian drug should not be prescribed prophylactically

- anxiolytic of choice if patient hallucinating, paranoid, or in agitated delirium.

Haloperidol versus chlorpromazine

- less sedative
- less anticholinergic effects
- less cardiovascular effects
- more potent anti-emetic
- more extrapyramidal reactions.

Therapeutic guidelines

Haloperidol is available in solution, capsule (0.5 mg), tablet (1.5, 5, 10, 20 mg) and parenteral forms.

Anti-emetic (for chemical/toxic causes of vomiting)

- 1.5 mg stat and nocte is standard for vomiting induced by morphine
- 3–5 mg nocte if smaller dose not effective
- 5–30 mg nocte (or in divided dosage) for vomiting induced by chemotherapy and in some patients with hypercalcaemia or uraemia.

Antipsychotic

- 1.5–3 mg stat and nocte in the elderly
- 5 mg stat and nocte in the younger patient or if poor response in the elderly
- 10–30 mg nocte (or in divided dosage) if poor response.

Anxiolytic

- 5 mg stat and nocte
- 10–20 mg nocte (or in divided dosage) if poor response.

Hyoscine

Hyoscine (scopolamine) is an anticholinergic with smooth muscle relaxant (antispasmodic) and antisecretory properties. It is available as *hydrobromide* and *butylbromide* (Buscopan) salts. The latter is a quaternary salt and does not cross the blood-brain barrier. Unlike hyoscine *hydrobromide*, hyoscine *butyl-bromide* does not cause drowsiness, nor does it have a central anti-emetic action.

General comments

- hyoscine *butylbromide* is poorly absorbed PO. By this route it is of use only in intestinal colic

- repeated administration of hyoscine *hydrobromide* leads to cumulation and may result paradoxically in an agitated delirium. If this occurs, add diazepam or midazolam.

Preparations

Hyoscine butylbromide

- PO 10 mg
- SC 20 mg.

Hyoscine hydrobromide

- SL 0.3 mg (Quick Kwell)
- SC 0.4 mg, 0.6 mg
- transdermal patch 0.5 mg over 3 days.

Therapeutic guidelines

Injections of hyoscine *butylbromide* are cheaper than hyoscine *hydrobromide* and should generally be used in preference. The main indications are

- death rattle
- inoperable bowel obstruction (*see* p.92).

Hyoscine *hydrobromide* by any route and hyoscine *butylbromide* SC can also be used in other situations where an anticholinergic may be beneficial, e.g. sialorrhoea.

Despite a plasma halflife of about 8 h, the duration of antisecretory effect after a single dose is only about 1 h (*butylbromide*) and 2 h (*hydrobromide*). Thus, hyoscine is best given as a transdermal patch or by continuous SC infusion.

Anticholinergic effects

'dry as a bone,
blind as a bat,
red as a beet,
hot as a hare,
mad as a hatter'

Several drugs used in palliative care have anticholinergic (antimuscarinic) properties (Table 4.22).

Table 4.22   Anticholinergic drugs used in palliative care

Belladonna alkaloids
  atropine
  hyoscine
	Antihistamines
	  chlorphenamine
	  cyclizine
	  dimenhydrinate
	  promethazine

Glycopyrronium	

Neuroleptics
  butyrophenones
  (haloperidol, droperidol)
  phenothiazines
	Antispasmodics
	  mebeverine
	  oxybutynin
	  propantheline

Tricyclic antidepressants	

Anticholinergic effects may be a limiting factor in symptom management. The concurrent use of two anticholinergic drugs should be avoided, if possible. A list of anticholinergic effects is given in Table 4.23.

Table 4.23   Anticholinergic effects

Visual

Mydriasis
Loss of accommodation   } blurred vision

Cardiovascular

Palpitations
Extrasystoles   } also related to norepinephrine potentiation and
Arrhythmias   a quinidine-like action

Gastro-intestinal

Dry mouth
Heartburn (reduced tone in lower oesophageal sphincter)
Constipation

Urinary tract

Hesitancy of micturition
Retention of urine

PART FIVE

Final Thoughts

When all's said and done
Professional carers have needs too

When all's said and done

Caring for the dying is full of paradoxes. One general practitioner wrote, 'I have looked after several patients who have died at home. I still find it extremely harrowing but very rewarding.'

Another doctor said to a patient's wife as he left the house, 'I don't know why I keep visiting, I never do anything.' To which the wife replied, 'Oh, Doctor Smith, don't say that! If only you knew the difference your visits make to us'.

Palliative care developed as a reaction to the attitude, spoken or unspoken, that 'there is nothing more that we can do for you' with the inevitable consequence for the patient and family of a sense of abandonment, hopelessness and despair. It was stressed that this was never true – there is always something that can be done. Even so, there are times when the doctor or nurse *feels* that he/she has nothing to offer. In this circumstance one is thrown back on who one is as an individual. Sheila Cassidy has illustrated this in a series of sketches (Figures 5.1–5.4).

> 'Slowly, I learn about the importance of powerlessness.
> I experience it in my own life and I live with it in my work.
> The secret is not to be afraid of it – not to run away.
> The dying know we are not God.
> All they ask is that we do not desert them.'[46]

When there is nothing to offer except ourselves, a belief that life has meaning and purpose helps to sustain the carer. However, to speak glibly of this to a patient who is in despair is cruel. At such times, actions speak louder than words. By what is done, the essential message is conveyed:

> 'You matter because you are you. You matter to the last moment of your life, and we will do all we can not only to help you die peacefully, but to live until you die.'[47]

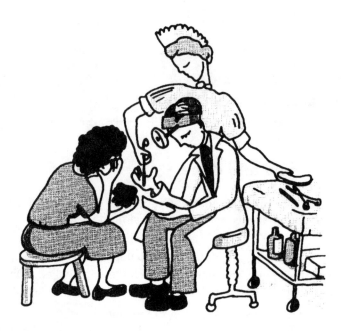

Figure 5.1 This shows the doctor, armed with his competence and his instruments and protected by his aide.[46] (Figures 5.1 to 5.4 are reproduced with permission from Cassidy S (1988) *Sharing the darkness*. DLT.)

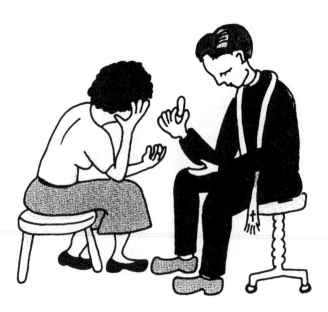

Figure 5.2 A priest performing his sacramental ministry. Here we see him wearing his stole and clerical collar protected by having a role to play and a ritual to perform.[46]

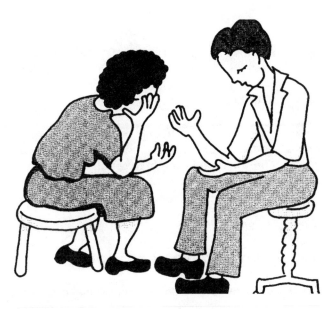

Figure 5.3   A patient meeting with either doctor or clergyman when he has exhausted the physical aspects of his ministry. He is left with his hands empty – but with his resources of counselling still available.[46]

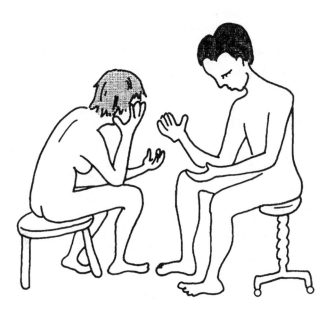

Figure 5.4   Both patient and carer stripped of their resources, present to each other, naked and empty handed, as two human beings.[46]

As someone observed:

'Those who have the strength and the love to sit with a dying patient in the silence that goes beyond words will know that this moment is neither frightening nor painful, but a peaceful cessation of the functioning of the body.

Watching a peaceful death of a human being reminds us of a falling star, one of the millions of lights in a vast sky that flares up for a brief moment only to disappear into the endless night forever.'[48]

Professional carers have needs too

Palliative care places many stresses on the professional carer. These include

- coping with the failure of medical cure
- repeated exposure to the death of people with whom we have formed a relationship
- involvement in emotional conflicts
- absorption of the anger expressed by patients and families
- role-blurring in multiprofessional teamwork
- personal idealism
- challenges to personal belief systems.

The following are prerequisites for self-care[49]

- love
- self-esteem
- a body image you accept
- a wish to develop creativity
- imagination
- flexibility
- humour

- compassion
- a capacity to accept mistakes and the ability to correct them
- a mind ready to take challenges.

> 'Caring is an ongoing creative process. If creativity is arrested or stopped, caring and hope are not possible. You have to restore creativity in order to restore hope.'[49]

A range of strategies helps to preserve emotional and physical health and avoid 'burnout'

- work as a team:
    shared decisions and responsibility
    mutual support and respect
- good communication within the team
- good resources and support services
- realistic goals
- be open to receive support from your patients
- adequate off-duty/food/rest
- time for recreation:
    hobbies
    spiritual refreshment.

Sometimes it is helpful to have the support of an outside professional counsellor, clinical psychologist or psychotherapist. There are many opportunities for personal growth within the challenges of palliative care. These challenges can be welcomed despite often being painful

- facing one's own mortality
- facing one's own limitations personally and professionally
- sharing control
- learning to be with patients, not just doing things for them
- facing challenges to one's own beliefs
- dealing honestly with personal emotions, e.g. anger, grief, hurt.

References

1   Wood CB (1984) In: CJH Van den Velde and PH Sugarbaker (eds) *Liver metastases*. Martinus Nijhoff, Dordrecht. pp 47–54.
2   Pettingale KW *et al.* (1985) Mental attitudes to cancer: an additional prognostic factor. *Lancet.* **i**: 750.
3   Frank A (1991) *At the will of the body: reflections on illness*. Houghton Mifflin, Boston.
4   Calman KC (1984) Quality of life in cancer patients – an hypothesis. *Journal of Medical Ethics.* **10**: 124–127.
5   Van Dam FSAM *et al.* (1984) Evaluating 'quality of life' in cancer clinical trials. In: ME Buyse *et al.* (eds) *Cancer clinical trials: methods and practice*. Oxford University Press, Oxford. pp 26–43.
6   Twycross RG (1987) Quality before quantity – a note of caution. *Palliative Medicine.* **1**: 65–72.
7   Cohen SR and Mount BM (1992) Quality of life in terminal illness: defining and measuring subjective well-being in the dying. *Journal of Palliative Care.* **8** (3): 40–45.
8   Gillon R (1994) Medical ethics: four principles plus attention to scope. *British Medical Journal.* **309**: 84–188.
9   Lunt B and Neale C (1987) A comparison of hospice and hospital: care goals set by staff. *Palliative Medicine.* **1**: 136–148.
10 Herth K (1990) Fostering hope in terminally-ill people. *Journal of Advanced Nursing.* **15**: 1250–1259.
11 Simpson MA (1979) *The facts of death*. Prentice-Hall, Englewood Cliffs, New Jersey.
12 Parkes CM (1972) Accuracy of predictions of survival in later stages of cancer. *British Medical Journal.* **ii**: 29–33.
13 Spiritual Care Working Group (1994) Sir Michael Sobell House, Oxford.
14 Kubotera T (1988) Personal communication.
15 Speck P (1984) *Being there: pastoral care in time of illness*. SPCK, London.
16 Department of Health (1991) *The patient's charter*. HMSO, London.
17 Gatrad AR (1994) Muslim customs surrounding death, bereavement, postmortem examinations, and organ transplants. *British Medical Journal.* **309**: 521–523.
18 Green J (1989) Hinduism. *Nursing Times.* **85** (6): 50–51.
19 Green J (1989) Buddhism. *Nursing Times.* **85** (9): 40–41.
20 Allingham M (1957) *The tiger in the smoke*. Penguin, Harmondsworth.
21 Campbell AB Quoted in: O'Toole D (1987) *Healing and growing through grief*. Blue Cross and Blue Shield, Michigan.
22 O'Toole D (1987) *Healing and growing through grief*. Blue Cross and Blue Shield, Michigan.
23 Parkes CM (1986) *Bereavement: studies of grief in adult life*. (2nd edn) Pelican, London.
24 Worden JW (1991) *Grief counselling and grief therapy*. (2nd edn) Tavistock, London.
25 Le Poidevin S Unpublished material.

26   Stroebe M (1994) Helping the bereaved to come to terms with loss: what does bereavement research have to offer. *Proceedings of the First St George's Conference 'Bereavement and Counselling'.* St George's Hospital Conference Unit, London.

27   Parkes CM (1990) Risk factors in bereavement: implications for the prevention and treatment of pathologic grief. *Psychiatric Annals.* **20**: 308–313.

28   Osterweiss M, Solomon F and Morris G (eds) (1984) *Bereavement reactions: consequences and care.* National Academy Press, Washington.

29   Raphael B (1977) Preventive intervention with the recently bereaved. *Archives of General Psychiatry.* **34**: 1450–1454.

30   Office of National Statistics, 1991 census.

31   Yaniv H (1994) Personal communication.

32   International Association for the Study of Pain Task Force on Taxonomy (1994) *Classification of chronic pain.* (2nd edn) IASP Press, Seattle.

33   Grond S *et al.* (1996) Assessment of cancer pain: a prospective evaluation in 2266 cancer patients referred to a pain service. *Pain.* **64**: 107–114.

34   World Health Organization (1986) *Cancer pain relief.* WHO, Geneva.

35   Guth B *et al.* (1996) Therapeutic doses of meloxicam do not inhibit platelet aggregation in man. *Rheumatology in Europe.* **25** (Suppl 1): Abs. 443.

36   Hanks G *et al.* (1996) Morphine in cancer pain: modes of administration. *British Medical Journal.* **312**: 823–826.

37   Ebert B *et al.* (1995) Ketobemidone, methadone and pethidine are noncompetitive N-methyl-D-Aspartate (NMDA) antagonists in the rat cortex and spinal cord. *Neuroscience Letters.* **187**: 165–168.

38   Bruera E *et al.* (1996) Opioid rotation in patients with cancer pain. *Cancer.* **78**: 852–857.

39   Twycross R and Lack SA (1986) *Control of Alimentary Symptoms in Far-Advanced Cancer.* Churchill Livingstone, Edinburgh.

40   Nelson KA *et al.* (1993) Assessment of upper gastrointestinal motility in the cancer-associated dyspepsia syndrome (CADS). *Journal of Palliative Care.* **9** (1): 27–31.

41   Krebs HB and Goplerud DR (1987) Mechanical intestinal obstruction in patients with gynecologic disease: A review of 368 patients. *American Journal of Obstetrics and Gynecology.* **157**: 577–583.

42   Davis C *et al.* (1996) Single dose randomised controlled trial of nebulised morphine in patients with cancer related breathlessness. *Palliative Medicine.* **10**: 64–65.

43   De Ruysscher D *et al.* (1996) Treatment of intractable hiccup in a terminal cancer patient with nebulized saline. *Palliative Medicine.* **10**: 166–167.

44   Brigham B and Bolin T (1992) High dose nifedipine and fludrocortisone for intractable hiccups. *The Medical Journal of Australia.* **157**: 70.

45   Sanger G and Twycross R (1996) Making sense of emesis, pruritus, 5HT & 5HT3 receptor antagonists. *Progress in Palliative Care.* **4**: 7–8.

46   Cassidy S (1988) *Sharing the darkness.* Darton, Longman and Todd, London. pp 61–64.

47   Saunders C Unpublished talk.

48   Kubler-Ross E (1969) *On death and dying.* Tavistock, London.

49   Bild R (1994) Personal communication.

Further reading

Specific

Twycross R (1995) Symptom Management in Advanced Cancer. Radcliffe Medical Press, Oxford.

Twycross RG (1994) *Pain relief in advanced cancer.* Churchill Livingstone, Edinburgh.

Stedeford A (1994) *Facing death: patients, families and professionals.* (2nd edn) Sobell Publications, Oxford.

Doyle D, Hanks GW and MacDonald N (eds) (1997) *Oxford textbook of palliative medicine.* (2nd edn) Oxford University Press, Oxford.

General

Barraclough J (1994) *Cancer and emotion.* John Wiley, Chichester.

Cassidy S (1988) *Sharing the darkness.* Darton, Longman and Todd, London.

Frank A (1991) *At the will of the body: reflections on illness.* Houghton Mifflin, Boston.

Frankl V (1959) *Man's search for meaning.* Simon and Shuster, New York.

Hill S (1974) *In the springtime of the year.* Penguin Books, London.

Lewis CS (1961) *A grief observed.* Faber and Faber, London.

Peck SM (1990) *The road less travelled: a new psychology of love, traditional values and spiritual growth.* Arrow Books, London.

Working Party Report (1991) *Mud and stars. The impact of hospice experience on the church's ministry of healing.* Sobell Publications, Oxford.

Index